No gall-bladder Diet Cookbook Guide

300 recipes for enjoy the healthy food before and after the gallbladder removal treatment

BRADY F. ROOTS

1

Table of Contents

SOUP AND STEWS 93

BROTHS, CONDIMENT AND SEASONING MIX 106

DESSERTS 125

21 days meal plan

Day	Breakfast	Lunch	Dinner
1	Oatmeal	Chicken wrap	Grilled salmon with asparagus
2	Scrambled eggs	Turkey chili	Shrimp scampi with zucchini noodles
3	Greek yogurt with granola	Beef stir-fry with broccoli	Baked chicken with sweet potatoes
4	Breakfast burrito	Lentil soup	Grilled pork chops with green beans
5	Cottage cheese with fruit	Tuna salad	Broiled tilapia with spinach salad
6	Protein smoothie	Grilled chicken with quinoa	Beef and mushroom stroganoff
7	Avocado toast	Turkey and cheese sandwich	Baked salmon with roasted carrots
8	Banana pancakes	Vegetable stir-fry with tofu	Turkey meatballs with spaghetti
9	Scrambled eggs with cheese	Chicken Caesar salad	Grilled sirloin steak with asparagus
10	Greek yogurt with honey	Lentil and vegetable stew	Baked chicken with roasted potatoes
11	Breakfast wrap	Chickpea salad	Shrimp and vegetable stir-fry

12	Protein oatmeal	Tomato soup	Grilled pork chops with zucchini
13	Cottage cheese with nuts	Chicken and vegetable stir-fry	Broiled tilapia with green beans
14	Green smoothie	Turkey chili	Beef and broccoli stir-fry
15	Bagel with cream cheese	Tuna and white bean salad	Baked salmon with roasted asparagus
16	Scrambled eggs with veggies	Grilled chicken with brown rice	Turkey meatloaf with sweet potatoes
17	Greek yogurt with fruit	Lentil soup	Grilled sirloin steak with broccoli
18	Breakfast burrito	Chickpea and vegetable stir-fry	Broiled tilapia with roasted veggies
19	Protein smoothie	Turkey and cheese sandwich	Beef and mushroom stir-fry
20	Avocado toast	Lentil and vegetable stew	Baked chicken with green beans
21	Banana pancakes	Chicken Caesar salad	Grilled salmon with zucchini noodles

introduction

The gallbladder is a small organ located under the liver, on the right side, it is pear-shaped and its main function is to collect and store bile, the liquid produced by the liver, yellowish in color and which is used for the proper digestion of fats. Therefore, this vesicle of the digestive system is crucial when it comes to being able to process fats to make use of and discard what is needed. Some people for various reasons may have to undergo an operation called cholecystectomy, in which this organ is removed due to health issues. It is very common that many questions arise about this situation and one of the most common, for example, is what to eat without a gallbladder.

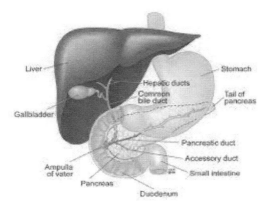

How to live without a gallbladder

Yes, you can live without a gallbladder, since although it plays an important role in the proper functioning of the body, this organ is not vital in itself.Those who have undergone a cholecystectomy, whether for chronic cholecystitis or other causes, spend a few days with low bile deposits, since they will only have available what has been stored in the small intestine until, little by little, it will begin to reach the duodenum directly from the liver, which can cause an excess of this liquid in the intestine. Therefore, of this liquid will not be sufficient for the digestion of fats and, therefore, if this type of food is ingested, digestive problems. The most common effects are nausea, vomiting, indigestion, gas and flatulence, bloating, diarrhea and colic. This recovery time usually lasts between 2 and 3 weeks, then little by little the food is reincorporated into the diet and you can live normally again.

In the event that there is an excess accumulation of bile in the small intestine, it will begin to move to and be absorbed by the large intestine, and an excess of bile salts may be produced in the large intestine and cause irritable bowel syndrome and diarrhea.

There are also many people who wonder if no gallbladder becomes fat or thin, and the truth is that, due to the reduction of fat and other factors, to weight loss and in some cases there are those who have difficulty in gaining weight afterwards.

In summary, after a gallbladder removal surgery it is necessary to adjust the diet and incorporate some foods slowly, over days or weeks. In fact, 95% of those who have surgery return to eating completely normally in a short time.

What can I eat if I have no gallbladder - recommended foods

<u>What can you eat after gallbladder surgery or cholecystectomy?</u> This is the main question and the truth is that you have to start by eliminating fat or eating very low fat foods, for example vegetable fats are generally better accepted after a cholecystectomy. These are the recommended foods if you do not have a gallbladder:

- Herbal teas and teas, such as green tea and chamomile tea
- Low-fat dairy products, whether milk, cheese or yogurt
- Legumes without skin and in moderation
- Pasta
- Rice
- Toast and crackers
- Fruits such as berries, apples, pears, peaches, etc.
- Vegetables, except those that are difficult to digest and flatulent
- White or lean fish
- Lean meats
- The only fatty foods allowed: olive or seed oil, preferably raw or well-boiled, never fried.

Prohibited or inadvisable foods after a cholecystectomy

Apart from the foods mentioned above, you must take into account the foods prohibited after a gallbladder operation, to eliminate them from the diet or, if the doctor indicates it, consume the right amounts so as not to suffer damage but take advantage of their nutrients.

- chocolate
- Coffee
- whole milk
- Fast food
- refined carbohydrates
- hydrogenated fats
- Fried and processed foods
- Fatty meats, such as sausages
- butter
- Blue fish and shellfish
- Eggs, especially the yolk
- Hard-skinned legumes
- Spicy and sauces
- Flatulent vegetables such as cauliflower, cabbage or artichokes
- olives
- Very fatty nuts such as hazelnuts and walnuts

7 Golden Secret Rules

You can do many things if you want to keep your kidneys healthy and have them functioning correctly. Here are seven secret golden rules that you can keep in mind for ensuring the proper functioning of your kidneys:

#1 Fitness Exercise

It is essential to ensure that you are moving your body and doing some form of exercise. Regarding the kidneys, it is not only crucial but also necessary to do some form of exercise. It is because it helps in preventing obesity from occurring. When a person is obese, and he or she then develops diabetes, the kidneys become strained. With exercise, the body can undergo some form of activity, which helps ensure the functioning and health of the kidneys.

#2 Regular Glycemic Check-Up

One of the most incredible things you can do to keep your kidneys healthy is to have your blood glucose, cholesterol, triglycerides, and uric acid levels checked regularly. Lowering these levels will certainly help in maintaining the essential health of your kidneys.

#3 Decrease Salt Amount

Although eating little salt wouldn't harm your kidneys, you must decrease the amount of salt you intake if you suffer from hypertension. Do you know that the kidneys are responsible for getting rid of any extra salt from your body? However, if you have different high blood pressure, then the kidneys will have a more challenging time getting rid of this extra salt. The kidneys are responsible for ridding your body of any excess salt, which is higher than the blood level in your body. You should also determine the sodium in your diet, which you can do by checking the food labels on your consuming foods. You should also avoid taking excess medicine, which contains sodium.

#4 Drink Water

Your body needs a specific or exact amount of water to function correctly and to keep calm. It is advisable to maintain your body hydrated at all times. Drink water or other liquids at least four times a day. At least 8-10 glasses of water are what you are supposed to drink every day. Water in itself can help you a lot if you want to keep your kidneys healthy.

#5 Don't Smoke

Smoking does affect the kidneys. Heavy smokers would be aware of this. If you want to maintain and keep your kidneys healthy, avoid smoking cigarettes at all costs. It is essential to understand that nicotine is what can damage all organs, including the kidneys. You should say no to smoking and keep your kidneys healthy.

#6 Eating Healthy Foods Plus Checking Weight Regularly

Eating healthy is the key to a healthy and fit body. You need to consume healthy foods that can help you beat kidney or any other kinds of diseases. Enjoying healthy foods at least once a day is what will help you keep your kidneys healthy. Include many fresh fruits and vegetables in your diet, and avoid oily, junk, processed foods.

You need to keep track of your weight and make sure that you check it regularly. Your weight needs to be in a healthy range. You can check your value in the morning and record in a diary before going to bed. You need to check your weight daily or on time and take note of the readings. Avoid gaining weight as this would undoubtedly put a lot of pressure on the kidneys.

#7 Keep the Kidney Warm (Hot Water Bag)

One of the best methods that have always been used and recommended by all kinds of doctors and medical practitioners are hot water bags. They can help in curing a lot of kidney problems and keeping them away. When kept in an affected area, hot water bags can help fix a lot of kidney-related questions. You need to keep them for a period of fifteen to twenty minutes. It would help in controlling all the pain away from the affected area. Also, please keep them in a clean room. Ensure that you do not place your bags in places where they may be exposed to dirt and bacteria.

For those people searching for recipes and renal diet guides to help you on the way to better kidneys' performance and overall well-being, this is it. We hope you will enjoy the renal diet recipes — let the benefits begin

13 Pillars f no Gall-bladder lifestyle
1. Avoid most, nut, and seed oils, including canola, sunflower, corn, grapeseed, and soybean oil, which now account for around 10% of our calories. Small quantities of expeller or cold-pressed nut and seed oils, such as sesame, macadamia, and walnut, can be used as condiments or flavorings. Avocado oil is suitable for cooking at higher temperatures.
2. Limit or exclude dairy. Dairy isn't good for most people, so I suggest avoiding it, with the exception of kefir, yogurt, ghee, Fat free butter or coconut spread, Instead of cow dairy, try goat or sheep dairy. Also, go organic and grass-fed whenever possible.
3. Consider meat and animal products as a side dish, or as I like to refer to them, "condi-meat," rather than the main course. Meat should be a side dish, with vegetables taking center stage. Per meal, servings should be no more than 4 to 6 ounces. I usually prepare three or four vegetable side dishes at a time.
4. Consume low-mercury fish that has been sustainably raised or harvested. Choose low-mercury and low-toxin seafood such as sardines, herring, anchovies, and wild-caught salmon if you're eating fish (all of which have high omega-3 and low mercury levels).
5. Stay away from gluten. Wheat can only be eaten if you are not gluten-intolerant, and even then, only on special occasions.
6. Avoid sugar all costs. That means avoiding sugar, starch, and refined carbohydrates, all of which cause an increase in insulin output. Consider sugar all of its types as a once-in-a-while indulgence, something we consume in moderation. People should think of it as a recreational drug, I tell them. It's something you do for fun now and then, but it's not something you eat every day.
7. Eat predominantly plant-based foods. Vegetables can occupy more than half of your plate, as we learned earlier. The better the hue, the darker it is. The greater the range, the better. Stop starchy vegetables as far as possible. In moderation (12 cups per day), winter squashes and sweet potatoes are perfect. There aren't enough potatoes! Even though French fries are America's most common vegetable, they don't count.
8. Taking it easy on the fruits. This is where there might be some misunderstanding. only low-sugar including berries, while vegan advocates advise eating all fruit. Many of my patients seem to feel happier when they stick to low-glycemic fruits and treat themselves to the rest. Stick to bananas, kiwis, and watermelon, and avoid oranges, melons, and other similar fruits. Consider dried fruit to be sweets, and use it sparingly.
9. Avoid pesticides, antibiotics, hormones, and genetically modified crops. Additionally, there are no pesticides, oils, preservatives, dyes, artificial sweeteners, or other potentially harmful ingredients. You should not eat an ingredient if you do not have it in your kitchen for cooking. Anyone for polysorbate 60, red dye 40, and sodium stearoyl lactylate (a.k.a. Twinkie ingredients)?
10. Consume gluten-free whole grains in moderation. They also increase blood sugar and have the ability to cause autoimmunity. A grain- and bean-free diet can be crucial for type 2 diabetics, as well as those with autoimmune disease or digestive disorders, in treating and even reversing their illness.
11. Just eat beans once in a while. The best legume is lentils. Big, starchy beans should be avoided. Beans have a high fiber, protein, and mineral content. However, for some people, they cause digestive issues, and the lectins and phytates in them can inhibit mineral absorption. If you have diabetes, a high-bean diet will cause blood blood spikes.

12. Get your solution checked so you can adapt it to your unique needs. What is effective for one individual might not be effective for another. This is what I mean when I say that everyone can eventually work with a functionally qualified nutritionist to personalize their diet even further with the right tests.
13. Stay away from booze and coffee.

Breakfast and Smoothies

Apple Turnover

Preparation Time: 10 minutes
Cooking Time: 15 minutes
Servings: 8
Ingredients:
For the turnovers:

- ½ tsp. cinnamon powder
- All-purpose flour
- ½ cup of stevia or aspartame
- 1 tbsp. almond flour
- 1 frozen puff pastry
- 4 peeled, cored, and diced baking apples.

For the egg wash:
- 2 tbsp water
- 1 whisked egg white

Directions:
1. For the filling, combine almond flour, cinnamon powder, stevia or aspartame until these resemble a coarse meal. Toss in diced apples until well coated. Set aside.
2. On your floured working surface, roll out the puff pastry until ¼ inch thin. Slice into 8 pieces of 4" x 4" squares. Divide the prepared apples into 8 equal portions, then spoon on individual puff pastry squares. Fold in half diagonally. Press edges to seal.
3. Place each filled pastry on a baking tray lined with parchment paper. Make sure there is ample space between pastries. Freeze within 20 minutes or until ready to bake.
4. Preheat oven to 400°F for 10 minutes. Brush frozen pastries with egg wash. Put in the hot oven, and cook within 12 to 15 minutes, or until they turn golden brown all over. Remove, then cool slightly for easier handling. Place 1 apple turnover on a plate. Serve warm.

Nutrition:
Calories 285
Carbs 35.75g
Fat 14.78g
Protein 3.81g
Potassium 151 mg
Sodium 86 mg
Phosphorus 43.4mg

Summer Squash and Apple Soup

Preparation time: 10 minutes
Cooking time: 40 minutes
Servings: 4
Ingredients:

- 1 cup non-dairy milk
- ½ tsp. cumin
- 3 cups unsalted vegetable broth
- 1 ½ tsp. Grated ginger
- 1 tbsp. olive oil
- 1 lb. peeled summer squash
- 2 diced apples
- ¾ tsp. curry powder

Directions:
1. Set the oven to 375 °F. Cut out a sheet of aluminum foil that is big enough to wrap the summer squash. Once covered, bake for 30 minutes.
2. Remove the wrapped summer squash from the oven and set aside to cool. Once cooled, remove the aluminum foil, remove the seeds, and peel.
3. Dice the summer squash, then place it in a food processor. Add non-dairy milk. Blend until smooth. Transfer to a bowl and set aside.
4. Place a soup pot over medium flame and heat through. Put the olive oil, then swirl to coat.
5. Sauté the onion until tender, then add the diced apple, spices, and broth, then boil. Once boiling, reduce to a simmer and let simmer for about 8 minutes.
6. Turn off, and let it cool slightly. Once cooled, pour the mixture into the food processor and blend until smooth.

7. Pour the pureed apple mixture back into the pot, then stir in the summer squash mixture. Mix well, then reheat to a simmer over medium flame. Serve.

Nutrition:
Calories 240
Protein 2.24g
Fat 8g
Carbs 40g
Potassium 376 mg
Sodium 429 mg
Phosphorus 0g

Roasted Pepper Soup

Preparation time: 10 minutes
Cooking time: 30 minutes
Servings: 4
Ingredients:
- 2 cups unsalted vegetable broth
- ½ cup chopped carrots
- 2 large red peppers
- ¼ cup julienned sweet basil
- 2 minced garlic cloves
- ½ cup chopped celery
- 2 tbsps. Olive oil
- ½ cup chopped onion
- ½ cup almond milk

Directions:
1. Place the oven at 375°F. Put onions on a baking sheet. Add the red peppers beside the mixture. Drizzle some of the olive oil over everything and toss well to coat.
2. Roast for 20 minutes, or until peppers are tender and skins are wilted. Chop the roasted red peppers and set aside.
3. Place a pot over medium-high flame and heat through. Put the olive oil and swirl to coat.
4. Place the carrot, celery, and garlic into the pot and sauté until carrot and celery are tender. Add the chopped roasted red peppers. Mix well.

5. Put in the vegetable broth plus almond milk. Increase to high flame and bring to a boil. Once boiling, reduce to a simmer. Simmer, uncovered, for 10 minutes.
6. If desired, blend the soup using an immersion blender until the soup has reached a desired level of smoothness. Reheat over medium flame. Add the basil and stir to combine. Serve.

Nutrition:
Calories 320
Protein 1.3g
Fat 25g
Carbs 20g
Potassium 249 mg
Sodium 45 mg
Phosphorus 66.33 g

Assorted Fresh Fruit Juice

Preparation Time:5 minutes
Cooking Time:0 minutes,
Servings:1
Ingredients:
- 1 roughly chopped apple
- ¼ cup halved frozen grapes
- 1 cup ice shavings

Directions:
1. Add all ingredients into the blender. Process until smooth. Pour equal portions into glasses. Serve immediately.

Nutrition:
Calories 112
Protein 1.16g
Potassium 367 mg
Sodium 3 mg
Fat 0.5g
Carbs 25.8g
Phosphorus 17.4mg

Raspberry and Pineapple Smoothie

Preparation Time: 5 minutes

Cooking Time: 15 seconds
Servings: 4
Ingredients:

- ½ cup crushed Ice
- 1 chopped small overripe banana piece
- 8 oz. rinsed and drained pineapple tidbits
- ½ cup frozen raspberries

Directions:
1. Except for cashew nuts and stevia, combine remaining ingredients in a deep microwave-safe bowl. Stir.
2. Microwave on the highest setting for about 5 to 15 seconds, then stop the cooking process before milk bubbles out of the bowl.
3. Carefully remove the bowl from the microwave. Cool slightly for easier handling. Stir in stevia if using. Sprinkle cashew nuts.

Nutrition:
Protein 3.1g
Potassium 749 mg
Sodium 4 mg
Calories 360
Fat 1g
Carbs 90g
Phosphorus 106.2mg

Fast Asparagus

Servings: 3 | Prep: 5m | Cooks: 10m | Total: 15m
INGREDIENTS
1 pound asparagus
1 teaspoon Cajun seasoning
DIRECTIONS
Preheat oven to 425 degrees F (220 degrees C).
Snap the asparagus at the tender part of the stalk.
Arrange spearsin one layer on a baking sheet.
Spray lightly with nonstick spray; sprinkle with the Cajun seasoning.
Bake in the preheated oven until tender, about 10 minutes.

NUTRITION FACTS
Calories: 32 | Carbohydrates: 6.3g | Fat: 0.2g | Protein: 3.4g | Cholesterol: 0mg

Olive Oil and Sesame Asparagus

Preparation Time: 5 minutes
Cooking Time: 5 minutes
Servings: 1
Ingredients:

- ½ tbsp. olive oil
- 2 cups sliced asparagus
- ½ cup water
- ½ tsp. sesame seeds
- 1/8 tsp. crushed red pepper flakes

Directions:
1. In a large skillet, boil the water. Place in the asparagus. Allow boiling for 2 minutes. Reduce heat, then cook for another 5 minutes. Drain asparagus and place on a plate. Set aside.
2. Meanwhile, heat the olive oil. Tip in asparagus and red pepper flakes. Sauté for 3 minutes. Remove from heat. Drizzle in more olive oil and sprinkle sesame seeds before serving.

Nutrition:
Calories 122
Protein 6.19g
Potassium 547 mg
Sodium 9 mg
Fat 7g
Carbs 11g
Phosphorus:37mg

Blueberries Mint French Toast

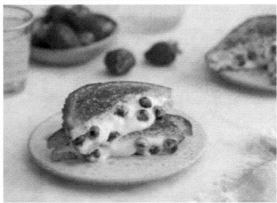

Preparation Time: 10 minutes
Cooking Time: 12 minutes
Servings: 2
Ingredients:
- Two spoon of coconut spread
- ¼ teaspoon mint
- ¼ cup of soy milk
- 1/8 cup blueberries
- 2 slices whole bread

Directions:
1. In a bowl, mix egg, soy milk, and mint. Add blueberries to the mixture. On medium-high heat, heat a nonstick pan. Soak bread slices in mixture and place on the pan. When the underside becomes brown, flip the bread and cook another side. Cut and serve.

Nutrition:
Calories 214
Fat 15g,
Sodium 165mg
Carbohydrate 15.3g
Protein 6.5g
Potassium 246mg
Phosphorus 114 g

Red Grapes Smoothie Bowl

Preparation Time: 10 minutes
Cooking Time: 12 minutes
Servings: 2
Ingredients:
- 1 cup red grapes
- 2 tablespoons whey protein powder
- 1/4 cup Greek yogurt, plain, non-fat
- 1/3 cup unsweetened almond milk
- 2 medium strawberries
- 5 raspberries
- 2 teaspoons shredded almond

Directions:
1. Place red grapes in a blender and blend on low for 1 minute. Add protein powder, yogurt, and almond milk. Blend to a soft-serve consistency. Scrape sides of the blender as needed. Scoop mixture into a bowl. Top with sliced strawberries, fresh raspberries, and almond flakes.

Nutrition:
Calories 320
Fat 12.8g,
Sodium 72mg
Carbohydrate 28.1g
Protein 26.8g
Potassium 370mg
Phosphorus 174 mg

Apple Tea Smoothie

Preparation Time: 35 minutes
Cooking Time: 5 minutes
Servings: 2
Ingredients:
- 1 cup unsweetened rice milk
- 1 teabag
- 1 apple, peeled, cored, and chopped
- 2 cups ice

Directions:
1. Heat the rice milk in a saucepan over low heat for 5 minutes or until steaming. Remove the milk and put it in the tea bag to steep.

2. Let the milk cool in the refrigerator with the tea bag for 30 minutes. Then remove the teabag, and squeeze gently to release all the flavor. Place the milk, apple, and ice in a blender and blend until smooth. Pour into 2 glasses and serve.

Nutrition:
Calories: 88
Fat: 0g
Carb: 19g
Phosphorus: 74mg
Potassium: 92mg
Sodium: 47mg
Protein: 1g

Blueberry-Pineapple Smoothie

Preparation Time: 15 minutes
Cooking Time: 0 minutes
Servings: 2
Ingredients:
- 1 cup frozen blueberries
- 1/2 cup pineapple chunks
- 1/2 cup English cucumber
- 1/2 apple
- 1/2 cup water

Directions:
1. Put the pineapple, blueberries, cucumber, apple, and water in a blender and blend until thick and smooth. Pour into 2 glasses and serve.

Nutrition:
Calories: 87
Fat: g
Carb: 22g
Phosphorus: 28mg
Potassium: 192mg
Sodium: 3mg
Protein: 0g

Festive Berry Parfait

Preparation Time: 60 minutes

Cooking Time: 0 minutes
Servings: 4
Ingredients:
- 1 cup vanilla rice milk, at room temperature
- 1/2 cup plain cream cheese, room temperature
- 1 tbsp granulated stevia or aspartame
- 1/2 tsp ground cinnamon
- 1 cup crumbled meringue cookies
- 2 cups fresh blueberries
- 1 cup sliced fresh strawberries

Directions:
1. Mix the milk, cream cheese, sugar, and cinnamon until smooth in a small bowl. Into 4 (6-ounce) glasses, spoon ¼ cup of crumbled cookie at the bottom of each.
2. Spoon ¼ cup of the cream cheese mixture on top of the cookies. Top the cream cheese with ¼ cup of the berries.
3. Repeat in each cup with the cookies, cream cheese mixture, and berries. Chill in the refrigerator for 1 hour and serve.

Nutrition:
Calories: 243
Fat: 1g
Carb: 33g
Phosphorus: 84mg
Potassium: 189mg
Sodium: 145mg
Protein: 4g

Mixed-Grain Hot Cereal

Preparation Time: 10 minutes
Cooking Time: 25 minutes
Servings: 4
Ingredients:
- 2 1/4 cups water
- 1 1/4 cups vanilla rice milk
- 6 tbsp uncooked bulgur
- 2 tbsp uncooked whole buckwheat
- 1 cup sliced apple

- 6 tbsp plain uncooked couscous
- 1/2 tsp ground cinnamon

Directions:
1. Heat the water and milk in a saucepan over medium heat. Boil, then add the bulgur, buckwheat, and apple.
2. Adjust the heat to low and simmer, occasionally stirring until the bulgur is tender, about 20 to 25 minutes.
3. Remove saucepan, then put the couscous and cinnamon and stir. Let the saucepan stand, covered, within 10 minutes. Fluff the cereal with a fork. Serve.

Nutrition:
Calories: 159
Fat: 1g
Carb: 34g
Phosphorus: 130mg
Potassium: 116mg
Sodium: 33mg
Protein: 4g

Cinnamon-Nutmeg Blueberry Muffins

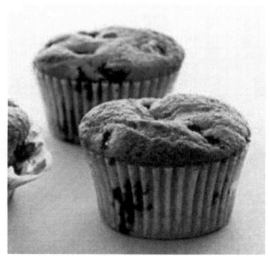

Preparation Time: 15 minutes
Cooking Time: 30 minutes
Servings: 12

Ingredients:
- 2 cups unsweetened rice milk
- 1 tbsp apple cider vinegar
- 3 1/2 cups all-purpose flour
- 1 cup granulated sugar
- 1 tbsp baking soda substitute
- 1 tsp ground cinnamon
- 1/2 tsp ground nutmeg
- pinch ground ginger
- 1/2 cup canola oil
- 2 tbsp pure vanilla extract
- 2 1/2 cups fresh blueberries

Directions:
1. Preheat the oven to 375F.
2. Mix the rice milk and vinegar in a small bowl. Set aside within 10 minutes. Mix the sugar, flour, baking soda, cinnamon, nutmeg, plus ginger in a large bowl.
3. Put the oil plus vanilla into the milk batter and stir to blend. Put the milk batter to the dry fixing and stir until combined.
4. Fold in the blueberries, then put the muffin batter evenly into the cups. Bake the muffins within 25 to 30, or until golden and a toothpick inserted comes out clean. Cool for 15 minutes and serve.

Nutrition:
Calories: 331
Fat: 11g
Carb: 52g
Phosphorus: 90mg
Potassium: 89mg
Sodium: 35mg
Protein: 6g

Fruit and Cheese Breakfast Wrap

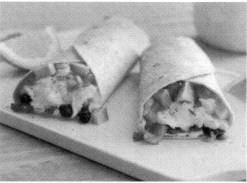

Preparation Time: 10 minutes
Cooking Time: 0 minutes
Servings: 2
Ingredients:

- 6 flour tortillas, 6-inch
- 2 tbsp coconut spread
- 1 apple,1 avocado , 2 kiwis and sliced thinly
- 1 tbsp honey

Directions:
1. Place both tortillas on a clean work surface and spread 1 tbsp of coconut spread on each tortilla, leaving half an inch around the edges.
2. Put all the fruit slices on coconut , besides the center of the tortilla on the side closest to you, leaving about 1 ½ inch on each side and two inches on the bottom.
3. Put honey over the apples lightly. Fold the left, then the right edges of the tortillas into the middle, laying the edge on the apples.
4. Taking the tortilla edge, fold it on the fruit, then the side pieces. Roll the tortilla, creating a snug wrap. Repeat it with the second tortilla. Serve.

Nutrition:
Calories: 188
Fat: 6g
Carb: 33g
Phosphorus: 73mg
Potassium: 136mg
Sodium: 177mg

Protein: 4g

Eggless Pancake
Preparation Time: 15 minutes

Cooking Time: 20 minutes
Servings: 2
Ingredients:
1 Cup All Purpose Flour
1 Teaspoon Sugar
1/4 Teaspoon Ground Cinnamon
2 Teaspoons Baking Powder
1/4 Teaspoon Salt
1 Cup Milk (I Used 2%)
1 Tablespoon Vegetable Oil
1 Tablespoon Water
1 Teaspoon Vanilla Extract
2 Table spoons Butter
Directions:
1. Whisk together the dry ingredients.
2. In a liquid measuring mug, measure 1 cup milk. To that add the vegetable oil, water and vanilla extract.
3. Stir in the wet ingredients to the dry ingredients. Do not over-mix. Lumps are perfectly fine. Set aside for a couple of minutes.
4. Heat a griddle at medium-high heat. Once the pan is hot add the butter and let it melt.
5. Add the melted butter to the pancake batter and return the pan to the stove. Mix the butter into the batter.
6. When the pan is hot enough, pour a ladleful of batter on the pan for each pancake. Cook until bubbles appear on the face of the pancake.
7. Carefully flip the pancake and cook until its golden brown

Nutrition:
Calories: 161
Fat: 1g

Carb: 30g
Phosphorus: 73mg
Potassium: 106mg
Sodium: 79mg
Protein: 7g

Berry Shake

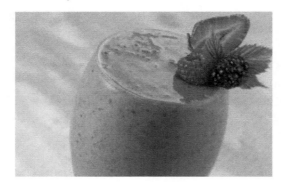

Preparation time: 5 minutes
Cooking time: 0 minutes
Servings: 1
Ingredients:
- ½ cup whole milk yogurt
- ¼ cup raspberries
- ¼ cup blackberry
- ¼ cup strawberries, chopped
- 1 tablespoon cocoa powder
- 1 ½ cups of water

Directions:
1. Blend all fixing in your blender until you have a smooth and creamy texture. Serve chilled and enjoy!

Nutrition:
Calories: 255
Fat: 19g
Carbohydrates: 20g
Protein: 6g
Sodium 80.5 mg
Potassium 360.6 mg
Phosphorus 141.7mg

Berry Smoothie

Preparation Time: 4 minutes
Cooking Time: 0 minute
Servings: 2
Ingredients:
- ¼ cup of frozen blueberries
- ¼ cup of frozen blackberries
- 1 cup of unsweetened almond milk
- 1 teaspoon of vanilla bean extract
- 3 teaspoons of flaxseed
- 1 scoop of chilled Greek yogurt
- Stevia as needed

Directions:
1. Mix everything in a blender and emulsify. Pulse the mixture four-times until you have your desired thickness. Pour the mixture into a glass. Enjoy!

Nutrition:
Calories: 221
Fat: 9g
Protein: 21g
Carbohydrates: 10g
Sodium 85 mg
Phosphorus 45 mg
Potassium 139 mg

Berry and Almond Smoothie

Preparation Time: 10 minutes
Cooking Time: 0 minute
Servings: 4
Ingredients:
- 1 cup of blueberries, frozen
- 1 whole banana
- ½ a cup of almond milk
- 1 tablespoon of almond Fat free butter or coconut spread
- water as needed

Directions:

1. Add the listed ingredients to your blender and blend well until you have a smoothie-like texture. Chill and serve. Enjoy!

Nutrition:
Calories: 321
Fat: 11g
Carbohydrates: 55g
Protein: 5g
Sodium 161.7mg
Potassium: 753.7mg
Phosphorus 145 mg

Mango and Pear Smoothie

Preparation Time: 10 minutes
Cooking Time: 0 minute
Servings: 1
Ingredients:
- 1 ripe mango, cored and chopped
- ½ mango, peeled, pitted, and chopped
- 1 cup kale, chopped
- ½ cup plain Greek yogurt
- 2 ice cubes

Directions:
1. Add pear, mango, yogurt, kale, and mango to a blender and puree. Add ice, then blend until a smooth texture is achieved. Serve and enjoy!

Nutrition:
Calories: 293
Fat: 8g
Carbohydrates: 53g
Protein: 8g
Sodium 29.4 mg
Potassium 632.3 mg
Phosphorus 63.4 mg

Blackberry and Apple Smoothie

Preparation Time: 5 minutes
Cooking Time: 0 minute
Servings: 2
Ingredients:

- 2 cups frozen blackberries
- ½ cup apple cider
- 1 apple, cubed
- 2/3 cup non-fat lemon yogurt

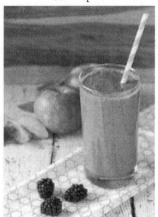

Directions:
1. Add the listed components to your blender and blend until smooth. Serve chilled!

Nutrition:
Calories: 200
Fat: 10g
Carbohydrates: 14g
Protein 2g
Phosphorus 5 mg
Potassium 199.4 mg
Sodium 63 mg

Minty Cherry Smoothie

Preparation Time: 5 minutes
Cooking Time: 0 minute
Servings: 2
Ingredients:
- ¾ cup cherries
- 1 teaspoon mint
- ½ cup almond milk
- ½ cup kale
- ½ teaspoon fresh vanilla

Directions:

1. Wash and cut cherries, take the pits out. Add cherries to the blender. Pour almond milk. Wash the mint and put two sprigs in a blender.
2. Separate the kale leaves from the stems. Put kale in a blender. Press vanilla bean and cut lengthwise with a knife.
3. Scoop out your desired amount of vanilla and add it to the blender. Blend until smooth. Serve chilled and enjoy!

Nutrition:
Calories: 200
Fat: 10g
Carbohydrates: 14g
Protein 2g
Phosphorus 220 mg
Potassium 674.2 mg
Sodium 226.1 mg

Fruit Smoothie

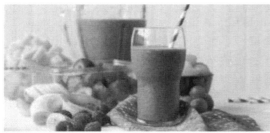

Preparation Time: 10 minutes
Cooking Time: 0 minute
Servings: 1
Ingredients:
- 1 cup spring-mix salad blend
- 2 cups of water
- 3 medium blackberries, whole
- 1 packet Stevia, optional
- 1 tablespoon coconut flakes shredded and unsweetened
- 2 tablespoons pecans, chopped
- 1 tablespoon hemp seed
- 1 tablespoon sunflower seed

Directions:
1. Add the ingredients all together into a blender. Blend on high until smooth and creamy. Enjoy your smoothie

Nutrition:
Calories: 385
Fat: 34g
Carbohydrates: 16g
Protein: 6.9g
Phosphorus 150 mg
Potassium 230 mg
Sodium 80 mg

Green Minty Smoothie

Preparation Time: 10 minutes
Cooking Time: 0 minute
Servings: 1
Ingredients:
- 1 stalk celery
- 2 cups of water
- 2 ounces almonds
- 1 packet Stevia
- 2 mint leaves

Directions:
1. In a blender, add all the ingredients. Blend well until a smooth and creamy texture is achieved. Serve chilled and enjoy!

Nutrition:
Calories: 417
Fat: 43g
Carbohydrates: 10g
Protein: 5.5g
Phosphorus 48 mg
Potassium 783.2 mg
Sodium 35.7 mg

Gut Cleansing Smoothie

Preparation Time: 10 minutes
Cooking Time: 0 minute
Servings: 1
Ingredients:

- 1 ½ tablespoons coconut oil, unrefined
- ½ cup plain full-fat yogurt
- 1 tablespoon chia seeds
- 1 serving aloe Vera leaves
- ½ cup frozen blueberries, unsweetened
- 1 tablespoon hemp hearts
- 1 cup of water
- 1 scoop Pinnaclife prebiotic fiber

Directions:
1. Add listed ingredients to a blender. Blend well until a smooth and creamy texture is achieved. Serve chilled and enjoy!

Nutrition:
Calories: 409
Fat: 33g
Carbohydrates: 8g
Protein: 12g
Phosphorus 81 mg
Potassium 746.1 mg
Sodium 45.9 mg

Blueberry and Kale Mix

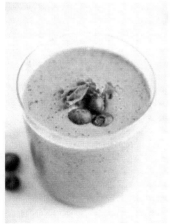

Preparation time: 5 minutes
Cooking time: 0 minutes
Servings: 1
Ingredients:

- ½ cup low-fat Greek Yogurt
- 1 cup baby kale greens
- 1 pack stevia
- 1 tablespoon MCT oil
- ¼ cup blueberries
- 1 tablespoon pepitas
- 1 tablespoon flaxseed, ground
- 1 ½ cups of water

Directions:
1. Put all fixing in a blender, blend until you have a smooth and creamy texture. Serve chilled!

Nutrition:
Calories: 307
Fat: 24g
Carbohydrates: 14g
Protein: 9g
Phosphorus 203 mg
Potassium 1 mg
Sodium 107.7 mg

Ginger Strawberry Shake

Preparation time: 5 minutes
Cooking time: 0 minutes
Servings: 1
Ingredients:

- 1 cup almond milk
- ½ teaspoon ginger powder
- 1 small stalk celery
- 1 cup spring salad mix
- 1 teaspoon sesame seeds
- 1 cup of water
- 1 pack Stevia

Directions:
1. Add listed ingredients to a blender. Blend it until you have a smooth smoothie. Serve chilled and enjoy!

Nutrition:
Calories: 475
Fat: 50g

Carbohydrates: 10g
Protein: 7g
Sodium 43.1 mg
Phosphorus 35.8 mg
Potassium 174.6 mg

Side and Snacks

VIETNAMESE FRESH SPRINGROLLS

Servings: 8 | Prep: 45m | Cooks: 5m | Total: 50m

INGREDIENTS

2 ounces rice vermicelli
1/4 cup water
8 rice wrappers (8.5 inch diameter)
2 tablespoons fresh lime juice
8 large cooked shrimp - peeled, deveined and cut in half
1 clove garlic, minced
1 1/3 tablespoons chopped fresh Thai basil
2 tablespoons white sugar
3 tablespoons chopped fresh mint leaves
1/2 teaspoon garlic chili sauce
3 tablespoons chopped fresh cilantro
3 tablespoons hoisin sauce
2 leaves lettuce, chopped
1 teaspoon finely chopped peanuts
4 teaspoons fish sauce

DIRECTIONS

Bring a medium saucepan of water to boil. Boil rice vermicelli 3 to5 minutes, or until al dente, and drain.

Fill a large bowl with warm water. Dip one wrapper into the hot water for 1 second to soften. Lay wrapper flat. In a row across the center, place 2 shrimp halves, a handful of vermicelli, basil, mint, cilantro and lettuce, leaving about 2 inches uncovered on each side.Fold uncovered sides inward, then tightly roll the wrapper, beginningat the end with the lettuce. Repeat with remaining ingredients.

In a small bowl, mix the fish sauce, water, lime juice, garlic, sugarand chili sauce.

In another small bowl, mix the hoisin sauce and peanuts.

Serve rolled spring rolls with the fish sauce and hoisin saucemixtures.

NUTRITION FACTS

Calories: 82 | Carbohydrates: 15.8g | Fat: 0.7g | Protein: 3.3g | Cholesterol: 11mg

Turkey Meatballs

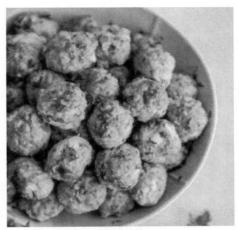

Preparation Time: 10 minutes
Cooking Time: 22 minutes
Servings: 12
Ingredients:

- 1 lb. ground turkey
- 1 large egg
- 1/4 cup bread crumbs
- 2 tablespoons onion, finely chopped
- 1 teaspoon garlic powder
- 1/2 teaspoons black pepper
- 1/4 cup canola oil
- 6 oz. grape jelly
- 1/4 cup chili sauce

Directions:

1. Start by tossing turkey meat along with all other ingredients in a bowl. Stir well until evenly mixed, then roll small meatballs out of this mixture. It will make as many as 48 meatballs.
2. Place these meatballs at the bottom of an Instant Pot. Whisk chili sauce with jelly in a

suitable bowl and cook it for 2 minutes in the microwave. Mix well, then add this batter to the meatballs.

3. Cook the saucy meatballs for 20 minutes approximately on Manual Mode at High pressure. Serve immediately.

Nutrition:
Calories 127
Fats 4 g
Sodium 121 mg
Carbs 14 g
Protein 9 g
Phosphorus 0 mg
Potassium 0 mg

Vegetable Corn Bread

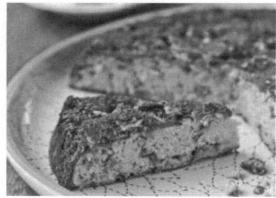

Preparation Time: 10 minutes
Cooking Time: 30 minutes
Servings: 6
Ingredients:
- 1 cup almond flour
- 1 cup plain cornmeal
- 1 tablespoon stevia or aspartame
- 2 teaspoons baking powder
- 1 teaspoon chili powder
- 1/4 teaspoons black pepper
- 1 cup rice milk, unenriched
- 1 egg
- 1 egg white
- 2 tablespoons canola oil
- 1/2 cup scallions, finely chopped
- 1/4 cup carrots, finely grated
- 1 garlic clove, minced

Directions:
1. Now begin mixing the flour with sugar, baking powder, cornmeal, pepper, and chili powder in a suitable mixing bowl. Pour in oil, milk, egg white, and egg. Stir well until it's smooth, then fold in garlic, carrots, and scallions.
2. Mix well evenly, then spread this batter in an 8-inch baking dish, greased with cooking spray. Put a cup of water into the bottom of the Instant Pot.
3. Place a steamer rack in the pot and set the baking dish over it. Cook the corn batter for 30 minutes approximately on Manual mode with High pressure until golden brown. Slice and serve fresh.

Nutrition:
Calories 188
Fats 5 g
Sodium 155 mg
Carbs 31 g
Protein 5 g
Phosphorus 98.6 mg
Potassium 138.6 mg

Chicken Peppers

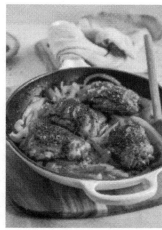

Preparation Time: 10 minutes
Cooking Time: 15 minutes
Servings: 6
Ingredients:
- 1 medium onion, chopped
- 12 fresh jalapenos peppers
- 12 fresh banana peppers
- 2 lbs. boneless, skinless chicken breast

Directions:
1. Slice the onion in quarters. Grease the rack of the instant with cooking spray. Discard the pepper's seed and chop them in half lengthwise.
2. Cut the chicken into 24 pieces, divide them into the peppers, and then top the chicken with an onion slice. Put a cup of water inside your Instant Pot.
3. Place the rack in the pot and arrange the peppers in the frame. Seal the lid and select the manual mode with high pressure for 15 minutes. Serve the peppers.

Nutrition:
Calories 115
Fats 7 g
Sodium 156 mg
Carbs 11 g
Protein 2 g

Potassium 556 mg
Phosphorus 146 mg

Buffalo Chicken Dip

Preparation Time: 10 minutes
Cooking Time: 7 minutes
Servings: 4
Ingredients:
- 4 ounces' cream cheese
- 1/2 cup bottled roasted red peppers
- 1 cup reduced-fat sour cream
- 4 teaspoons hot pepper sauce
- 2 cups cooked, shredded chicken

Directions:
1. Blend ½ cup of drained red peppers in a food processor until smooth. Now evenly mix cream cheese, sour cream, and 2 tablespoons Tabasco sauce with the bowl's peppers.
2. Toss in chicken; hot sauce, then transfers the mixture to the Instant Pot. Cook on high within 7 minutes. Serve.

Nutrition:
Calories 73
Fats 5 g
Sodium 66 mg
Carbs 2 g
Protein 5 g
Potassium 161 mg
Phosphorus 236 mg

Prosciutto-Wrapped Asparagus

Preparation Time: 10 minutes
Cooking Time: 3 minutes

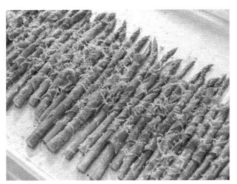

Servings: 4
Ingredients:

- 1lb thick Asparagus
- 8oz thinly sliced Prosciutto
- Black pepper to taste

Directions:
1. Put 1 cup of water inside your pot and place a rack over it. Take an asparagus spear and wrap it with a prosciutto slice.
2. Continue wrapping all the asparagus spears this way. Place the spears over the rack and then seal the lid.
3. Cook for 3 minutes on Manual mode at High pressure. Serve wrapped spears with black pepper on top. Enjoy.

Nutrition:
Calories 71
Fats 3 g
Sodium 96 mg
Carbs 1 g
Protein 10 g
Potassium 129 mg
Phosphorus 82.4 mg

Fat free butter or coconut spread & Garlic Mushrooms

Preparation Time: 10 minutes
Cooking Time: 20 minutes

Servings: 4
Ingredients:

- 2 tablespoons olive oil
- 1 lb. small button mushrooms
- 2 tablespoons Fat free butter or coconut spread
- 2 teaspoons minced garlic
- 1/2 teaspoons fresh thyme

Directions:
1. Start by preheating the Instant pot on Sauté mode. Add olive oil and mushrooms to the pool and sauté for 5 minutes.
2. Add garlic, thyme, and Fat free butter or coconut spread, then mix well to coat. Seal the pot's lid and cook for 15 minutes on Manual mode with high pressure. Serve.

Nutrition:
Calories 118
Fats 7 g
Sodium 166 mg
Carbs 12 g
Protein 2 g
Potassium 395.1 mg
Phosphorus 98 mg

Savory Collard Chips

Preparation Time: 5 minutes
Cooking Time: 20 minutes
Servings: 4
Ingredients:

- 1 bunch of collard greens
- 1 teaspoon of extra-virgin olive oil
- Juice of ½ lemon
- ½ teaspoon of garlic powder
- ¼ teaspoon of freshly ground black pepper

Directions:
1. Preheat the oven to 350°F. Line a baking sheet with parchment paper. Cut the collards into 2-by-2-inch squares and pat dry with paper towels.

2. Toss greens with the olive oil, lemon juice, garlic powder, and pepper in a large bowl. Put the dressing into the gardens, then massage using your hands until evenly coated.
3. Arrange the collards in a single layer on the baking sheet, and cook for 8 minutes. Flip and cook again within 8 minutes, until crisp. Remove from oven, let cool.

Nutrition:
Calories: 24
Fat: 1g
Carbohydrates: 3g
Protein: 1g
Phosphorus: 6mg
Potassium: 72mg
Sodium: 8mg

Roasted Red Pepper Hummus

Preparation Time: 10 minutes

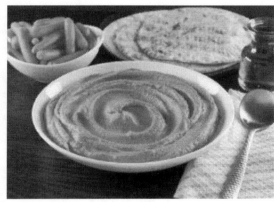

Cooking Time: 10 minutes
Servings: 8
Ingredients:
- 1 red bell pepper
- 1 can of chickpeas, drained
- Juice of 1 lemon
- 2 tablespoons of tahini
- 2 garlic cloves
- 2 tablespoons of extra-virgin olive oil

Directions:

1. Move the rack of the oven to the highest position. Heat the broiler to high. Core the pepper and cut it into three or four large pieces. Arrange them on a baking sheet, skin-side up.
2. Broil the peppers for 5 to 10 minutes, until the skins are charred. Remove from the oven, then transfer the peppers to a small bowl. Cover with plastic wrap and let them steam for 10 to 15 minutes, until cool enough to handle.
3. Peel the burnt skin off the peppers, and place the peppers in a blender. Add the chickpeas, lemon juice, tahini, garlic, and olive oil. Wait until smooth, then add up to 1 tablespoon of water to adjust consistency as desired.

Nutrition:
Calories: 103
Fat: 6g
Carbohydrates: 10g
Protein: 3g
Phosphorus: 58mg
Potassium: 91mg
Sodium: 72mg

Thai-Style Eggplant Dip

Preparation Time: 10 minutes
Cooking Time: 30 minutes
Servings: 4

Ingredients:
- 1 pound of Thai eggplant (or Japanese or Chinese eggplant)
- 2 tablespoons of rice vinegar
- 2 teaspoons of stevia or aspartame
- 1 teaspoon of low-sodium soy sauce
- 1 jalapeño pepper
- 2 garlic cloves
- ¼ cup of chopped basil
- Cut vegetables or crackers for serving

Directions:

1. Preheat the oven to 425°F to get it ready. Pierce every eggplant with a skewer or knife. Put on a rimmed baking sheet and cook within 30 minutes. Let cool, cut in half, and scoop out the flesh of the eggplant into a blender.
2. Add the rice vinegar, sugar, soy sauce, jalapeño, garlic, and basil to the blender. Process until smooth. Serve with cut vegetables or crackers.

Nutrition:
Calories: 40
Fat: 0g
Carbohydrates: 10g
Protein: 2g
Phosphorus: 34mg
Potassium: 284mg
Sodium: 47mg

Chicken Satay

Servings: 12 | Prep: 2h10m | Cooks: 20m | Total:2h40m | Additional: 10m
INGREDIENTS
2 tablespoons creamy peanut butter
2 tablespoons curry powder
1/2 cup soy sauce
2 cloves garlic, chopped
1/2 cup lemon or lime juice
1 teaspoon hot pepper sauce
1 tablespoon brown sugar
6 skinless, boneless chicken breast halves – cubed
DIRECTIONS
In a mixing bowl, combine peanut butter, soy sauce, lime juice, brown sugar, curry powder, garlic and hot pepper sauce. Place the chicken breasts in the marinade and refrigerate. Let the chicken marinate at least 2 hours, overnight is best.
Preheat a grill to high heat.

Weave the chicken onto skewers, then grill for 5 minutes per side.

NUTRITION FACTS
Calories: 162 | Carbohydrates: 4.1g | Fat: 3g | Protein: 28.8g |Cholesterol: 68mg

Coconut Pancakes

Preparation Time: 5 minutes
Cooking Time: 10 minutes
Servings: 2
Ingredients:
- 2 free-range egg whites
- 2 tbsp of all-purpose white flour
- 3 tbsp of coconut shavings
- 2 tbsp of coconut milk (optional)
- 1 tbsp of coconut oil

Directions:
1. Get a bowl and combine all the ingredients. Mix well until you get a thick batter. Heat a skillet on medium heat and heat the coconut oil.
2. Pour half the mixture to the pan's center, forming a pancake, and cook through for 3-4 minutes on each side. Serve with your choice of berries on the top.

Nutrition:
Calories: 177
Fat: 13g
Carbohydrates: 12g
Phosphorus: 37mg
Potassium: 133mg
Sodium: 133mg
Protein: 5g

Spiced Peaches

Preparation Time: 5 minutes

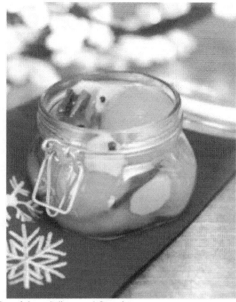

Cooking Time: 10 minutes

Servings: 2

Ingredients:

- 1 cup of canned peaches in their juices
- 1/2 tsp of cornstarch
- 1 tsp of ground cloves
- 1 tsp of ground cinnamon
- 1 tsp of ground nutmeg
- 1/2 lemon zest
- 1/2 cup of water

Directions:

1. Drain peaches. Combine water, cornstarch, cinnamon, nutmeg, ground cloves, and lemon zest in a pan on the stove. Heat on medium heat and add peaches. Boil, then adjust the heat and simmer for 10 minutes. Serve warm.

Nutrition:

Calories: 70

Fat: 1g

Carbohydrates: 18g

Phosphorus: 26mg

Potassium: 184mg

Sodium: 9mg

Protein: 1g

European Pancakes

Preparation Time: 5 minutes

Cooking Time: 20 minutes

Servings: 10

Ingredients:

- 2/3 cups of all-purpose flour
- 2 tbsp. of stevia or aspartame
- ½ tsp. of lemon zest
- 1 cup of low-fat milk
- ¼ tsp. of vanilla extract

Directions:

1. Mix flour, stevia , then whisk in the water and combine well. Put then the milk, vanilla, and lemon zest to the mix and whisk well.
2. Spray a small 8–10-inch pan with cooking spray and pour around 4 tbsp of the mixture and distribute evenly by tilting the pan from one side to another.
3. Cook until the batter or mixture is solid and light golden brown (around 50 seconds on each side). Flip. Repeat the process with the remaining batter.

Nutrition:

Calories: 74

Carbohydrate: 10g

Protein: 4g

Sodium: 39mg

Potassium: 73mg

Phosphorus: 73mg

Fat: 2g

Sandwich with Chicken Salad

Preparation Time: 10 minutes

Cooking Time: 10 minutes

Servings: 2

Ingredients:

- 2 bowls of cooked chicken
- 1/2 cup of low-fat mayonnaise
- 1/2 cup of green bell pepper
- 1 cup of pieces pineapple
- 1/3 cup of carrots
- 4 slices of flatbread
- 1/2 tsp of black pepper

Directions:
1. Prepare aside the diced chicken and drain pineapple, adding green bell pepper, black pepper, and carrots. Combine all in a bowl and refrigerate until chilled. Later on, serve the chicken salad on the flatbread. Enjoy!

Nutrition:
Calories: 345
Protein: 22g
Carbohydrate: 0g
Sodium: 395mg
Fat: 0g
Potassium: 330mg
Phosphorus: 165mg

Celery and Arugula Salad

Preparation Time: 10 minutes
Cooking Time: 0 minute
Servings: 4
Ingredients:
- 1 shallot, thinly sliced
- 3 celery stalks, slice into 1-inch pieces about ¼ inch thick
- 2 cups of loosely packed arugula
- 1 tablespoon of extra-virgin olive oil
- 2 tablespoons of white wine vinegar
- Freshly ground black pepper
- 2 tablespoons of grated Parmesan cheese

Directions:
1. In a medium bowl, toss the shallot, celery stalks, and arugula. In a small bowl, whisk the olive oil, vinegar, and pepper. Toss your salad with your dressing. Top with Parmesan cheese and serve.

Nutrition:
Calories: 45
Fat: 4g
Carbs: 1g
Protein: 1g
Phosphorus: 23mg
Potassium: 47mg
Sodium: 47mg

Baked Sweet potato sticks

Servings: 8 | Prep: 15m | Cooks: 40m | Total: 55m
INGREDIENTS
1 tablespoon olive oil
8 sweet potatoes, sliced lengthwise into quarters
1/2 teaspoon paprika
DIRECTIONS
Preheat oven to 400 degrees F (200 degrees C). Lightly grease abaking sheet.
In a large bowl, mix olive oil and paprika. Add potato sticks, andstir by hand to coat. Place on the prepared baking sheet.
Bake 40 minutes in the preheated oven
NUTRITION FACTS
Calories: 132 | Carbohydrates: 27g | Fat: 1.9g | Protein: 2.6g | Cholesterol: 0mg

Chicken, Charred Tomato, and Carrot Salad

Preparation Time: 10 minutes
Cooking Time: 30 minutes
Servings: 6
Ingredients:
- ¼ cup of lemon juice
- ½ tsp of chili powder
- 1 ½ lb. of boneless chicken breast
- 1 ½ lb. of a medium tomato
- 1 tsp of freshly ground pepper
- 1 tsp of sea salt
- 4 cups of Carrotflorets
- 5 tbsp of extra virgin olive oil, divided into 2 and 3 tablespoons

Directions:
1. Place the chicken in a skillet and add just enough water to cover the chicken. Bring to a simmer over high heat.
2. Reduce the heat once the liquid boils and cook the chicken thoroughly for 12 minutes. Once cooked, shred the chicken into bite-sized pieces.
3. On a large pot, bring water to a boil and add the broccoli. Cook for 5 minutes until slightly tender. Drain and rinse the Carrotusing cold water. Set aside.
4. Core the tomatoes and cut them crosswise. Discard the seeds and set the tomatoes cut-side down on paper towels. Pat them dry.
5. In a heavy skillet, heat the pan over high heat. Brush the slice sides of the tomatoes with olive oil and place them on the pan. Cook the tomatoes until the sides are charred. Set aside.
6. In the same pan, heat the remaining 3 tablespoon olive oil over medium heat. Stir the salt, chili powder, and pepper and stir for 45 seconds.
7. Pour over the lemon juice and remove the pan from the heat. Plate the broccoli, shredded chicken, and chili powder mixture dressing.

Nutrition:
Calories: 277
Carbs: 6g
Protein: 28g
Fat: 9g
Phosphorus: 292mg
Potassium: 719mg
Sodium: 560mg

Stuffed Artichokes

Preparation time: 10 minutes
Cooking time: 1 hour and 10 minutes
Servings: 4
Ingredients:
- 4 artichokes, stems cut off and hearts chopped
- 3 garlic cloves, minced
- 2 cups spinach, chopped
- 1 tablespoon coconut oil, melted
- 1 yellow onion, chopped
- 4 ounces shallots, chopped, cooked, and crumbled
- A pinch of black pepper

Directions:
1. Put artichokes in a large saucepan, add water to cover, bring to a boil over medium heat, cook for 30 minutes, drain them and leave them aside to cool down.
2. Heat-up a pan with the oil over medium-high heat, add onion, stir and cook for 10 minutes. Add spinach, stir, cook for 3 minutes, take off the heat and leave aside to cool down.
3. Put cooked shallots in your food processor, add artichoke insides as well and pulse well. Add this to spinach and onion mix and stir well.
4. Place artichoke cups on a lined baking sheet, stuff them with spinach mix, put in the oven at 375 F, then bake within 30 minutes. Divide the artichokes between plates and serve as a side dish.

Nutrition:
Calories 144
Fat 3.8g
Carbs 25.6g
Protein 6.9g
Phosphorus 172.3 mg
Potassium 254.9 mg
Sodium 368.7 mg

Ginger Cauliflower Rice

Preparation time: 10 minutes

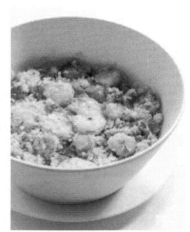

Cooking time: 10 minutes
Servings: 4
Ingredients:

- 5 cups cauliflower florets
- 3 tablespoons coconut oil
- 4 ginger slices, grated
- 1 tablespoon coconut vinegar
- 3 garlic cloves, minced
- 1 tablespoon chives, minced
- A pinch of sea salt
- Black pepper to taste

Directions:
1. Pulse the cauliflower using your food processor. Heat-up a pan with the oil over medium-high heat, add ginger, stir and cook for 3 minutes.

Nutrition:
Fat 0.5g
Carbs 20.8g
Protein 4.1g

Cauliflower and Leeks

Preparation time: 10 minutes
Cooking time: 20 minutes

2. Add cauliflower rice and garlic, stir and cook for 7 minutes. Add salt, black pepper, vinegar, chives, stir, cook for a few seconds more, divide between plates, and serve.

Nutrition:
Calories 125
Fat 10.4g
Carbs 79g
Protein 2.7g
Phosphorus 35 mg
Potassium 228.3 mg
Sodium 21.9 mg

Braised Cabbage

Preparation time: 10 minutes
Cooking time: 10 minutes
Servings: 4
Ingredients:

- 1 small cabbage head, shredded
- 2 tablespoons water
- A drizzle of olive oil
- 6 ounces shallots, cooked and chopped
- A pinch of black pepper
- A bit of sweet paprika
- 1 tablespoon dill, chopped

Directions:
1. Heat-up a pan with the oil over medium heat, add the cabbage and the water, stir and sauté for 5 minutes. Put the rest of the fixing, toss, cook for 5 minutes more, divide everything between plates, and serve as a side dish!

Calories 91
Phosphorus 37.7 mg
Potassium 268.4 mg
Sodium 250.9 mg
Servings: 4
Ingredients:

- 1 and ½ cups leeks, chopped
- 1 and ½ cups cauliflower florets
- 2 garlic cloves, minced

- 1 and ½ cups artichoke hearts
- 2 tablespoons coconut oil, melted
- Black pepper to taste

Directions:

1. Heat-up a pan with the oil over medium-high heat, add garlic, leeks, cauliflower florets, artichoke hearts, stir and cook for 20 minutes. Add black pepper, go, divide between plates and serve.

Nutrition:
Calories 192
Fat 6.9g
Carbs 35.1g

Protein 5.1g
Phosphorus 60.1 mg
Potassium 373.1 mg
Sodium 165.8 mg

Fish, Meat and Poultry

SPICY CHICKEN BREASTS

Servings: 4 | Prep: 15m | Cooks: 15m | Total: 30m

INGREDIENTS

2 1/2 tablespoons paprika
1 tablespoon dried thyme
2 tablespoons garlic powder
1 tablespoon ground cayenne pepper
1 tablespoon salt
1 tablespoon ground black pepper
1 tablespoon onion powder
4 skinless, boneless chicken breast halves

DIRECTIONS

In a medium bowl, mix together the paprika, garlic powder, salt, onion powder, thyme, cayenne pepper, and ground black pepper. Setaside about 3 tablespoons of this seasoning mixture for the chicken; store the remainder in an airtight container for later use (for seasoning fish, meats, or vegetables).

Preheat grill for medium-high heat. Rub some of the reserved 3tablespoons of seasoning onto both sides of the chicken breasts.

Lightly oil the grill grate. Place chicken on the grill, and cook for 6to 8 minutes on each side, until juices run clear.

NUTRITION FACTS
Calories: 173 | Carbohydrates: 9.2g | Fat: 2.4g | Protein: 29.2g | Cholesterol: 68mg

COD WITH ITALIAN CRUMBTOPPING
COD WITH ITALIAN CRUMBTOPPING

Cod with Italian Crumbtopping

Servings: 4 | Prep: 15m | Cooks: 10m | Total: 25m

INGREDIENTS

1/4 cup fine dry bread crumbs
1/8 teaspoon garlic powder
2 tablespoons grated Parmesan cheese
1/8 teaspoon ground black pepper
1 tablespoon cornmeal
4 (3 ounce) fillets cod fillets
1 teaspoon olive oil
1 egg white, lightly beaten
1/2 teaspoon Italian seasoning

DIRECTIONS

Preheat oven to 450 degrees F (230 degrees C). In a small shallow bowl, stir together the bread crumbs, cheese, cornmeal, oil, italian seasoning, garlic powder and pepper; set aside.

Coat the rack of a broiling pan with cooking spray. Place the cod on the rack, folding under any thin edges of the filets. Brush with theegg white, then spoon the crumb mixture evenly on top.

Bake in a preheated oven for 10 to 12 minutes or until the fishflakes easily when tested with a fork and is opaque all the way through.

NUTRITION FACTS
Calories: 131 | Carbohydrates: 7g | Fat: 2.9g | Protein: 18.1g | Cholesterol: 39mg

Shrimp Paella

Preparation time: 25 minutes
Cooking time: 10 minutes
Servings: 2
Ingredients:

- 1 cup cooked brown rice
- 1 chopped red onion
- 1 tsp. paprika
- 1 chopped garlic clove
- 1 tbsp. olive oil
- 6 oz. frozen cooked shrimp
- 1 deseeded and sliced chili pepper
- 1 tbsp oregano

Directions:

1. Warm-up olive oil in a large pan on medium-high heat. Add the onion and garlic and sauté for 2-3 minutes until soft. Now add the shrimp and sauté for a further 5 minutes or until hot through.
2. Now add the herbs, spices, chili, and rice with 1/2 cup boiling water. Stir until everything is warm, and the water has been absorbed. Plate up and serve.

Nutrition:
Calories 221
Protein 17 g
Carbs 31 g
Fat 8 g
Sodium 235 mg
Potassium 176 mg
Phosphorus 189 mg

Salmon & Pesto Salad

Preparation time: 5 minutes
Cooking time: 15 minutes
Servings: 2
Ingredients:
For the pesto:
- 1 minced garlic clove
- ½ cup fresh arugula
- ¼ cup extra virgin olive oil
- ½ cup fresh basil
- 1 tsp black pepper

For the salmon:
- 4 oz. skinless salmon fillet
- 1 tbsp coconut oil

Baked Fennel & Garlic Sea Bass

Preparation time: 5 minutes
Cooking time: 15 minutes
Servings: 2
Ingredients:
- 1 lemon
- ½ sliced fennel bulb

For the salad:
- ½ juiced lemon
- 2 sliced radishes
- ½ cup iceberg lettuce
- 1 tsp black pepper

Directions:
1. Prepare the pesto by blending all the fixing for the pesto in a food processor or grinding with a pestle and mortar. Set aside.
2. Add a skillet to the stove on medium-high heat and melt the coconut oil. Add the salmon to the pan. Cook for 7-8 minutes and turn over.
3. Cook within 3-4 minutes or until cooked through. Remove fillets from the skillet and allow to rest.
4. Mix the lettuce and the radishes and squeeze over the juice of ½ lemon. Shred the salmon using a fork and mix through the salad. Toss to coat and sprinkle with a little black pepper to serve.

Nutrition: Calories 221
Protein 13 g
Carbs 1 g
Fat 34 g
Sodium 80 mg
Potassium 119 mg
Phosphorus 158 mg

- 6 oz. sea bass fillets
- 1 tsp black pepper
- 2 garlic cloves

Directions:
1. Preheat the oven to 375°F. Sprinkle black pepper over the Sea Bass. Slice the fennel bulb and garlic cloves. Add 1 salmon fillet and half the fennel and garlic to one baking paper or tin foil sheet.

2. Squeeze in 1/2 lemon juices. Repeat for the other fillet. Fold and add to the oven for 12-15 minutes or until fish is thoroughly cooked through.
3. Meanwhile, add boiling water to your couscous, cover, and allow to steam. Serve with your choice of rice or salad.

Nutrition:
Calories 221
Protein 14 g
Carbs 3 g
Fat 2 g
Sodium 119 mg
Potassium 398 mg
Phosphorus 149 mg

Lemon, Garlic, Cilantro Tuna and Rice

Preparation time: 5 minutes
Cooking time: 0 minutes
Servings: 2
Ingredients:
- ½ cup arugula
- 1 tbsp extra virgin olive oil
- 1 cup cooked rice
- 1 tsp black pepper
- ¼ finely diced red onion
- 1 juiced lemon
- 3 oz. canned tuna
- 2 tbsp Chopped fresh cilantro

Directions:
1. Mix the olive oil, pepper, cilantro, and red onion in a bowl. Stir in the tuna, cover, then serve with the cooked rice and arugula!

Nutrition:
Calories 221
Protein 11 g
Carbs 26 g
Fat 7 g
Sodium 143 mg
Potassium 197 mg
Phosphorus 182 mg

Cod & Green Bean Risotto

Preparation time: 4 minutes
Cooking time: 40 minutes
Servings: 2
Ingredients:
- ½ cup arugula
- 1 finely diced white onion
- 4 oz. cod fillet
- 1 cup white rice
- 2 lemon wedges
- 1 cup boiling water
- ¼ tsp. black pepper
- 1 cup low-sodium chicken broth
- 1 tbsp extra virgin olive oil
- ½ cup green beans

Directions:
1. Warm-up oil in a large pan on medium heat. Sauté the chopped onion for 5 minutes until soft before adding in the rice and stirring for 1-2 minutes.
2. Combine the broth with boiling water. Add half of the liquid to the pan and stir. Slowly add the rest of the juice while continuously stirring for up to 20-30 minutes.
3. Stir in the green beans to the risotto. Place the fish on top of the rice, cover, and steam for 10 minutes.
4. Use your fork to break up the fish fillets and stir into the rice. Sprinkle with freshly ground pepper to serve and a squeeze of fresh lemon. Serve with the lemon wedges and the arugula.

Nutrition:
Calories 221
Protein 12 g
Carbs 29 g
Fat 8 g
Sodium 398 mg
Potassium 347 mg
Phosphorus 241 mg

Sardine Fish Cakes

Preparation Time: 10 minutes

Cooking Time: 10 minutes
Servings: 4

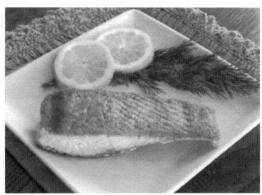

Ingredients:
- 11 oz sardines, canned, drained
- 1/3 cup shallot, chopped
- 1 teaspoon chili flakes
- ½ teaspoon salt
- 2 tablespoon wheat flour, whole grain
- 1 egg, beaten
- 1 tablespoon chives, chopped
- 1 teaspoon olive oil
- 1 teaspoon Fat free butter or coconut spread

Directions:
1. Put the Fat free butter or coconut spread in your skillet and dissolve it. Add shallot and cook it until translucent. After this, transfer the shallot to the mixing bowl.
2. Add sardines, chili flakes, salt, flour, egg, chives, and mix up until smooth with the fork's help. Make the medium size cakes and place them in the skillet. Add olive oil.
3. Roast the fish cakes for 3 minutes from each side over medium heat. Dry the cooked fish cakes with a paper towel if needed and transfer to the serving plates.

Nutrition:
Calories 221
Fat 12.2g
Fiber 0.1g
Carbs 5.4g

Protein 21.3 g
Phosphorus 188.7 mg
Potassium 160.3 mg
Sodium 452.6 mg

Cajun Catfish

Preparation Time: 10 minutes
Cooking Time: 10 minutes
Servings:4
Ingredients:
- 16 oz catfish steaks (4 oz each fish steak)
- 1 tablespoon Cajun spices
- 1 egg, beaten
- 1 tablespoon sunflower oil

Directions:
1. Pour sunflower oil into the skillet and preheat it until shimmering. Meanwhile, dip every catfish steak in the beaten egg and coat in Cajun spices.
2. Place the fish steaks in the hot oil and roast them for 4 minutes from each side. The cooked catfish steaks should have a light brown crust.

Nutrition:
Calories 263
Fat 16.7g
Fiber 0g
Carbs 0.1g
Protein 26.3g
Sodium 776 mg
Phosphorus 5 mg
Potassium 37.9 mg

4-Ingredients Salmon Fillet

Preparation Time: 5 minutes
Cooking Time: 25 minutes
 Servings:1
Ingredients:
- 4 oz salmon fillet
- ½ teaspoon salt
- 1 teaspoon sesame oil

- ½ teaspoon sage

Directions:
1. Rub the fillet with salt and sage. Put the fish in the tray, then sprinkle it with sesame oil. Cook the fish for 25 minutes at 365F. Flip the fish carefully onto another side after 12 minutes of cooking. Serve.

Nutrition:
Calories 191
Fat 11.6g
Fiber 0.1g
Carbs 0.2g
Protein 22g
Sodium 70.5 mg
Phosphorus 472 mg
Potassium 636.3 mg

Spanish Cod in Sauce

Preparation Time: 10 minutes
Cooking Time: 5 1/2 hours
Servings: 2
Ingredients:
- 1 teaspoon tomato paste
- 1 teaspoon garlic, diced
- 1 white onion, sliced
- 1 jalapeno pepper, chopped
- 1/3 cup chicken stock
- 7 oz Spanish cod fillet
- 1 teaspoon paprika
- 1 teaspoon salt

Directions:
1. Pour chicken stock into the saucepan. Add tomato paste and mix up the liquid until homogenous. Add garlic, onion, jalapeno pepper, paprika, and salt.
2. Bring the liquid to boil and then simmer it. Chop the cod fillet and add it to the tomato liquid. Simmer the fish for 10 minutes over low heat. Serve the fish in the bowls with tomato sauce.

Nutrition:

Calories 113
Fat 1.2g
Fiber 1.9g
Carbs 7.2g
Protein 18.9g
Potassium 659 mg
Sodium 597 mg
Phosphorus 18 mg

Salmon Baked in Foil with Fresh Thyme

Preparation Time: 10 minutes
Cooking Time: 30 minutes
Servings:4
Ingredients:
- 4 fresh thyme sprigs
- 4 garlic cloves, peeled, roughly chopped
- 16 oz salmon fillets (4 oz each fillet)
- ½ teaspoon salt
- ½ teaspoon ground black pepper
- 4 tablespoons cream
- 4 teaspoons Fat free butter or coconut spread
- ¼ teaspoon cumin seeds

Directions:
1. Line the baking tray with foil. Sprinkle the fish fillets with salt, ground black pepper, cumin seeds, and arrange them in the tray with oil.
2. Add thyme sprig on the top of every fillet. Then add cream, Fat free butter or coconut spread, and garlic. Bake the fish for 30 minutes at 345F. Serve.

Nutrition:
Calories 198
Fat 11.6g
Carbs 1.8g
Protein 22.4g
Phosphorus 425 mg
Potassium 660.9 mg
Sodium 366 mg

Poached Halibut in Orange Sauce

Preparation Time: 10 minutes
 Cooking Time: 10 minutes
Servings: 4
Ingredients:
- 1-pound halibut
- 1/3 cup Fat free butter or coconut spread
- 1 rosemary sprig
- ½ teaspoon ground black pepper
- 1 teaspoon salt
- 1 teaspoon honey
- ¼ cup of orange juice
- 1 teaspoon cornstarch

Directions:
1. Put Fat free butter or coconut spread in the saucepan and melt it. Add rosemary sprig. Sprinkle the halibut with salt and ground black pepper. Put the fish in the boiling Fat free butter or coconut spread and poach it for 4 minutes.
2. Meanwhile, pour orange juice into the skillet. Add honey and bring the liquid to boil. Add cornstarch and whisk until the liquid starts to be thick. Then remove it from the heat.
3. Transfer the poached halibut to the plate and cut it on 4. Place every fish serving in the serving plate and top with orange sauce.

Nutrition:
Calories 349
Fat 29.3g
Fiber 0.1g
Carbs 3.2g
Protein 17.8g
Phosphorus 154 mg
Potassium 388.6 mg
Sodium 29.3 mg

Fish En' Papillote

Preparation Time: 15 minutes
Cooking Time: 20 minutes
 Servings: 3

Ingredients:
- 10 oz snapper fillet
- 1 tablespoon fresh dill, chopped
- 1 white onion, peeled, sliced
- ½ teaspoon tarragon
- 1 tablespoon olive oil
- 1 teaspoon salt
- ½ teaspoon hot pepper
- 2 tablespoons sour cream

Directions:
1. Make the medium size packets from parchment and arrange them in the baking tray. Cut the snapper fillet into 3 and sprinkle them with salt, tarragon, and hot pepper.
2. Put the fish fillets in the parchment packets. Then top the fish with olive oil, sour cream, sliced onion, and fresh dill. Bake the fish for 20 minutes at 355F. Serve.

Nutrition:
Calories 204
Fat 8.2g
Carbs 4.6g
Protein 27.2g
Phosphorus 138.8 mg
Potassium 181.9 mg
Sodium 59.6 mg

Tuna Casserole

Preparation Time: 15 minutes
Cooking Time: 35 minutes
Servings:4
Ingredients:
- ½ cup Cheddar cheese, shredded
- 2 tomatoes, chopped
- 7 oz tuna filet, chopped
- 1 teaspoon ground coriander
- ½ teaspoon salt
- 1 teaspoon olive oil
- ½ teaspoon dried oregano

Directions:

1. Brush the casserole mold with olive oil. Mix up together chopped tuna fillet with dried oregano and ground coriander.
2. Place the fish in the mold and flatten well to get the layer. Then add chopped tomatoes and shredded cheese. Cover the casserole with foil and secure the edges. Bake the meal for 35 minutes at 355F. Serve.

Nutrition:
Calories 260
Fat 21.5g
Carbs 2.7g
Protein 14.6g
Phosphorus 153 mg
Potassium 311 mg
Sodium 600 mg

Fish Chili with Lentils

Preparation Time: 10 minutes
Cooking Time: 30 minutes
 Servings:4
Ingredients:
- 1 red pepper, chopped
- 1 yellow onion, diced
- 1 teaspoon ground black pepper
- 1 teaspoon Fat free butter or coconut spread
- 1 jalapeno pepper, chopped
- ½ cup lentils
- 3 cups chicken stock
- 1 teaspoon salt
- 1 tablespoon tomato paste
- 1 teaspoon chili pepper
- 3 tablespoons fresh cilantro, chopped
- 8 oz cod, chopped

Directions:
1. Place Fat free butter or coconut spread, red pepper, onion, and ground black pepper in the saucepan. Roast the vegetables for 5 minutes over medium heat.
2. Then add chopped jalapeno pepper, lentils, and chili pepper. Mix up the mixture well and add chicken stock and tomato paste. Stir

until homogenous. Add cod. Close the lid and cook chili for 20 minutes over medium heat.

Nutrition:
Calories 187
Fat 2.3g
Carbs 21.3g
Protein 20.6g
Phosphorus 50 mg
Potassium 281 mg
Sodium 43.8 mg

Chili Mussels

Preparation Time: 7 minutes
Cooking Time: 10 minutes
Servings:4
Ingredients:
- 1-pound mussels
- 1 chili pepper, chopped
- 1 cup chicken stock
- ½ cup milk
- 1 teaspoon olive oil
- 1 teaspoon minced garlic
- 1 teaspoon ground coriander
- ½ teaspoon salt
- 1 cup fresh parsley, chopped
- 4 tablespoons lemon juice

Directions:
1. Pour milk into the saucepan. Add chili pepper, chicken stock, olive oil, minced garlic, ground coriander, salt, and lemon juice.
2. Bring the liquid to boil and add mussels. Boil the mussel for 4 minutes or until they will open shells. Then add chopped parsley and mix up the meal well. Remove it from the heat.

Nutrition:
Calories 136
Fat 4.7g
Fiber 0.6g
Carbs 7.5g
Protein 15.3g
Phosphorus 180.8 mg

Potassium 312.5 mg
Sodium 319.6 mg

Beef and Chili Stew

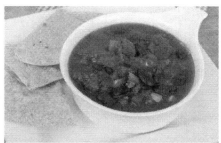

Preparation Time: 15 minutes
Cooking Time: 7 hours
Servings: 6
Ingredients:
- 1/2 medium red onion, sliced thinly
- 1/2 tablespoon vegetable oil
- 10ounce of flat-cut beef brisket, whole
- ½ cup low sodium stock
- ¾ cup of water
- ½ tablespoon honey
- ½ tablespoon chili powder
- ½ teaspoon smoked paprika
- ½ teaspoon dried thyme
- 1 teaspoon black pepper
- 1 tablespoon corn starch

Directions:
1. Throw the sliced onion into the slow cooker first. Add a splash of oil to a large hot skillet and briefly seal the beef on all sides.
2. Remove the beef, then place it in the slow cooker. Add the stock, water, honey, and spices to the same skillet you cooked the beef meat.
3. Allow the juice to simmer until the volume is reduced by about half. Pour the juice over beef in the slow cooker. Cook on low within 7 hours.
4. Transfer the beef to your platter, shred it using two forks. Put the rest of the juice into a medium saucepan. Bring it to a simmer.

5. Whisk the cornstarch with two tablespoons of water. Add to the juice and cook until slightly thickened.
6. For a thicker sauce, simmer and reduce the juice a bit more before adding cornstarch. Put the sauce on the meat and serve.

Nutrition:
Calories: 128
Protein: 13g
Carbohydrates: 6g
Fat: 6g
Sodium: 228mg
Potassium: 202mg
Phosphorus: 119mg

Beef and Three Pepper Stew

Preparation Time: 15 minutes
Cooking Time: 6 hours
Servings: 6
Ingredients:
- 10ounce of flat-cut beef brisket, whole
- 1 teaspoon of dried thyme
- 1 teaspoon of black pepper
- 1 clove garlic
- ½ cup of green onion, thinly sliced
- ½ cup low-sodium chicken stock
- 2 cups of water
- 1 large green bell pepper, sliced
- 1 large red bell pepper, sliced
- 1 large yellow bell pepper, sliced
- 1 large red onion, sliced

Directions:
1. Combine the beef, thyme, pepper, garlic, green onion, stock, and water in a slow cooker. Leave it all to cook on high for 4-5 hours until tender.
2. Remove the beef from the slow cooker and let it cool. Shred the beef meat using two forks, then discard any excess fat. Put the shredded beef meat back into the slow cooker.

3. Add the sliced peppers and the onion. Cook this on high heat for 40-60 minutes until the vegetables are tender.

Nutrition:
Calories: 132
Protein: 14g
Carbohydrates: 9g
Fat: 5g
Sodium: 179mg
Potassium: 390mg
Phosphorus: 141mg

Sticky Pulled Beef Open Sandwiches

Preparation Time: 15 minutes
Cooking Time: 5 hours
Servings: 5
Ingredients:
- ½ cup of green onion, sliced
- 2 garlic cloves
- 2 tablespoons of fresh parsley
- 2 large carrots
- 7ounce of flat-cut beef brisket, whole
- 1 tablespoon of smoked paprika
- 1 teaspoon dried parsley
- 1 teaspoon of brown stevia or aspartame
- ½ teaspoon of black pepper
- 2 tablespoon of olive oil
- ¼ cup of red wine
- 8 tablespoon of cider vinegar
- 3 cups of water
- 5 slices white bread
- 1 cup of arugula to garnish

Directions:
1. Finely chop the green onion, garlic, and fresh parsley. Grate the carrot. Put the beef in to roast in a slow cooker.
2. Add the chopped onion, garlic, and remaining ingredients, leaving the rolls, fresh parsley, and arugula to one side. Stir in the slow cooker to combine.

3. Cover and cook on low within 8 1/2 to 10 hours or on high for 4 to 5 hours until tender. Remove the meat from the slow cooker. Shred the meat using two forks.
4. Return the meat to the broth to keep it warm until ready to serve. Lightly toast the bread and top with shredded beef, arugula, fresh parsley, and ½ spoon of the broth. Serve.

Nutrition:
Calories: 273
Protein: 15g
Carbohydrates: 20g
Fat: 11g
Sodium: 308mg
Potassium: 399mg
Phosphorus: 159mg

Herby Beef Stroganoff and Fluffy Rice

Preparation Time: 15 minutes
Cooking Time: 5 hours
Servings: 6
Ingredients:
- ½ cup onion
- 2 garlic cloves
- 9ounce of flat-cut beef brisket, cut into 1" cubes
- ½ cup of reduced-sodium beef stock
- 1/3 cup red wine
- ½ teaspoon dried oregano
- ¼ teaspoon freshly ground black pepper
- ½ teaspoon dried thyme
- ½ teaspoon of saffron
- ½ cup almond milk (unenriched)
- ¼ cup all-purpose flour
- 1 cup of water
- 2 ½ cups of white rice

Directions:
1. Dice the onion, then mince the garlic cloves. Mix the beef, stock, wine, onion, garlic, oregano, pepper, thyme, and saffron in your slow cooker.

2. Cover and cook on high within 4-5 hours. Combine the almond milk, flour, and water. Whisk together until smooth.
3. Add the flour mixture to the slow cooker. Cook for another 15 to 25 minutes until the stroganoff is thick.
4. Cook the rice using the package instructions, leaving out the salt. Drain off the excess water. Serve the stroganoff over the rice.

Nutrition:
Calories: 241
Protein: 15g
Carbohydrates: 29g
Fat: 5g
Sodium: 182mg
Potassium: 206mg
Phosphorus: 151mg

Chunky Beef and Potato Slow Roast

Preparation Time:15 minutes
Cooking Time: 5-6 hours
Servings: 12
Ingredients:
- 3 cups of peeled potatoes, chunked
- 1 cup of onion
- 2 garlic cloves, chopped
- 1 ¼ pound flat-cut beef brisket, fat trimmed
- 2 cups of water
- 1 teaspoon of chili powder
- 1 tablespoon of dried rosemary

For the sauce:
- 1 tablespoon of freshly grated horseradish
- ½ cup of almond milk (unenriched)
- 1 tablespoon lemon juice (freshly squeezed)
- 1 garlic clove, minced
- A pinch of cayenne pepper

Directions:
1. Double boil the potatoes to reduce their potassium content. Chop the onion and the garlic. Place the beef brisket in a slow cooker.

Combine water, chopped garlic, chili powder, and rosemary.
2. Pour the mixture over the brisket. Cover and cook on high within 4-5 hours until the meat is very tender. Drain the potatoes and add them to the slow cooker.
3. Adjust the heat to high and cook covered until the potatoes are tender. Prepare the horseradish sauce by whisking together horseradish, milk, lemon juice, minced garlic, and cayenne pepper.
4. Cover and refrigerate. Serve your casserole with a dash of horseradish sauce on the side.

Nutrition:
Calories: 199
Protein: 21g
Carbohydrates: 12g
Fat: 7g
Sodium: 282mg
Potassium: 317
Phosphorus: 191mg

Spiced Lamb Burgers

Preparation Time: 10 minutes
Cooking Time: 20 minutes
Servings: 2
Ingredients:
- 1 tablespoon extra-virgin olive oil
- 1 teaspoon cumin
- ½ finely diced red onion
- 1 minced garlic clove
- 1 teaspoon harissa spices
- 1 cup arugula
- 1 juiced lemon
- 6-ounce lean ground lamb
- 1 tablespoon parsley
- ½ cup low-fat plain yogurt

Directions:
1. Preheat the broiler on medium to high heat. Mix the ground lamb, red onion, parsley, Harissa spices, and olive oil until combined.

2. Shape 1-inch thick patties using wet hands. Add the patties to a baking tray and place under the broiler for 7-8 minutes on each side. Mix the yogurt, lemon juice, and cumin and serve over the lamb burgers with arugula's side salad.

Nutrition:
Calories 306
Fat 20g
Carbs 10g
Phosphorus 269mg
Potassium 492mg
Sodium 86mg
Protein 23g

Pork Loins with Leeks

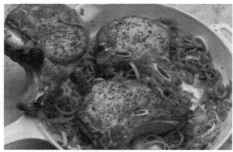

Preparation Time: 10 minutes
Cooking Time: 35 minutes
Servings: 2
Ingredients:
- 1 sliced leek
- 1 tablespoon mustard seeds
- 6-ounce pork tenderloin
- 1 tablespoon cumin seeds
- 1 tablespoon dry mustard
- 1 tablespoon extra-virgin oil

Directions:
1. Preheat the broiler to medium-high heat. In a dry skillet, heat mustard and cumin seeds until they start to pop (3-5 minutes). Grind seeds using a pestle and mortar or blender and then mix in the dry mustard.

2. Massage the pork on all sides using the mustard blend and add to a baking tray to broil for 25-30 minutes or until cooked through. Turn once halfway through.
3. Remove and place to one side, then heat-up the oil in a pan on medium heat and add the leeks for 5-6 minutes or until soft. Serve the pork tenderloin on a bed of leeks and enjoy it!

Nutrition:
Calories 139
Fat 5g
Carbs 2g
Phosphorus 278mg
Potassium 45mg
Sodium 47mg
Protein 18g

Chinese Beef Wraps

Preparation Time: 10 minutes
Cooking Time: 30 minutes
Servings: 2
Ingredients:
- 2 iceberg lettuce leaves
- ½ diced cucumber
- 1 teaspoon canola oil
- 5-ounce lean ground beef
- 1 teaspoon ground ginger
- 1 tablespoon chili flakes
- 1 minced garlic clove
- 1 tablespoon rice wine vinegar

Directions:
1. Mix the ground meat with the garlic, rice wine vinegar, chili flakes, and ginger in a bowl. Heat-up oil in a skillet over medium heat.
2. Put the beef in the pan and cook for 20-25 minutes or until cooked through. Serve beef mixture with diced cucumber in each lettuce wrap and fold.

Nutrition:

Calories 156
Fat 2g
Carbs 4 g
Phosphorus 1 mg
Sodium 54mg
Protein 14g
Potassium 0mg

Grilled Skirt Steak

Preparation Time: 15 minutes
Cooking Time: 8-9 minutes
Servings: 4
Ingredients:
- 2 teaspoons fresh ginger herb, grated finely
- 2 teaspoons fresh lime zest, grated finely
- ¼ cup of coconut stevia or aspartame
- 2 teaspoons fish sauce
- 2 tablespoons fresh lime juice
- ½ cup of coconut milk
- 1-pound beef skirt steak, trimmed and cut into 4-inch slices lengthwise
- Salt, to taste

Directions:
1. In a sizable sealable bag, mix all ingredients except steak and salt. Add steak and coat with marinade generously.
2. Fridge to marinate for about 4-12 hours. Preheat the grill to high heat. Grease the grill grate.
3. Remove steak from the refrigerator and discard the marinade. With a paper towel, dry the steak and sprinkle with salt evenly.
4. Cook the steak for approximately 3½ minutes. Flip the medial side and cook for around 2½-5 minutes or till the desired doneness.
5. Remove from the grill pan and keep the side for approximately 5 minutes before slicing. Cut it into desired slices and serve.

Nutrition:
Calories: 465
Fat: 10g

Carbohydrates: 22g
Protein: 37g
Phosphorus144.1 mg
Potassium277 mg
Sodium 816.7 mg

Spicy Lamb Curry

Preparation Time: 15 minutes
Cooking Time: 2 hours 15 minutes
Servings: 6-8
Ingredients:
- 4 teaspoons ground coriander
- 4 teaspoons ground coriander
- 4 teaspoons ground cumin
- ¾ teaspoon ground ginger
- 2 teaspoons ground cinnamon
- ½ teaspoon ground cloves
- ½ teaspoon ground cardamom
- 2 tablespoons sweet paprika
- ½ tablespoon cayenne pepper
- 2 teaspoons chili powder
- 2 teaspoons salt
- 1 tablespoon coconut oil
- 2 pounds boneless lamb, trimmed and cubed into 1-inch size
- Salt
- ground black pepper
- 2 cups onions, chopped
- 1¼ cups water
- 1 cup of coconut milk

Directions:
1. For spice mixture in a bowl, mix all spices. Keep aside. Season the lamb with salt and black pepper.
2. Warm oil on medium-high heat in a large Dutch oven. Add lamb and stir fry for around 5 minutes. Add onion and cook approximately 4-5 minutes.
3. Stir in the spice mixture and cook approximately 1 minute. Add water and coconut milk and provide some boil on high heat.

4. Adjust the heat to low and simmer, covered for approximately 1-120 minutes or until the lamb's desired doneness. Uncover and simmer for about 3-4 minutes. Serve hot.

Nutrition:
Calories: 466
Fat: 10g
Carbohydrates: 23g
Protein: 36g
Potassium 599 mg
Sodium 203 mg
Phosphorus 0mg

Lamb with Prunes
Preparation Time: 15 minutes
Cooking Time: 2 hours and 40 minutes
Servings: 4-6
Ingredients:
- 3 tablespoons coconut oil
- 2 onions, chopped finely
- 1 (1-inch) piece fresh ginger, minced
- 3 garlic cloves, minced
- ½ teaspoon ground turmeric
- 2 ½ pound lamb shoulder, trimmed and cubed into 3-inch size
- Salt
- ground black pepper
- ½ teaspoon saffron threads, crumbled
- 1 cinnamon stick
- 3 cups of water
- 1 cup prunes, pitted and halved

Directions:
1. In a big pan, melt coconut oil on medium heat. Add onions, ginger, garlic cloves, and turmeric and sauté for about 3-5 minutes. Flavor the lamb with salt plus black pepper evenly.
2. In the pan, add lamb and saffron threads and cook for approximately 4-5 minutes. Add cinnamon stick and water and produce to some boil on high heat.

3. Adjust to low and simmer, covered for around 1½-120 minutes or till the desired doneness of lamb. Stir in prunes and simmer for approximately 20-a half-hour. Remove cinnamon stick and serve hot.

Nutrition:
Calories: 393
Fat: 12g
Carbohydrates: 10g
Protein: 36g
Phosphorus 133.3 mg
Potassium 0.16 mg
Sodium 78 mg

Roast Beef
Preparation Time: 25 minutes
Cooking Time: 55 minutes
Servings: 3
Ingredients:
- Quality rump or sirloin tip roast
- Pepper & herbs

Directions:
1. Place in a roasting pan on a shallow rack. Season with pepper and herbs. Insert meat thermometer in the center or thickest part of the roast.
2. Roast to the desired degree of doneness. After removing from over for about 15 minutes, let it chill. In the end, the roast should be moister than well done.

Nutrition:
Calories 158
Protein 24 g
Fat 6 g
Carbs 0 g
Phosphorus 206 mg
Potassium 328 mg
Sodium 55 mg

Beef Brochettes
Preparation Time: 20 minutes

Cooking Time: 1 hour
Servings: 1
Ingredients:
- 1 ½ cups pineapple chunks
- 1 large sliced onion
- 2 pounds thick steak
- 1 sliced medium bell pepper
- 1 bay leaf
- ¼ cup of vegetable oil
- ½ cup lemon juice
- 2 crushed garlic cloves

Directions:
1. Cut beef cubes and place them in a plastic bag. Combine marinade ingredients in a small bowl. Mix and pour over beef cubes.
2. Seal the bag and refrigerate within 3 to 5 hours. Divide ingredients onion, beef cube, green pepper, pineapple. Grill about 9 minutes each side, serve.

Nutrition:
Calories 304
Protein 35 g
Fat 15 g
Carbs 11 g
Phosphorus 264 mg
Potassium 388 mg
Sodium 70 mg

Country Fried Steak

Preparation Time: 10 minutes
Cooking Time: 1 hour and 40 minutes
Servings: 3
Ingredients:
- 1 large onion
- ½ cup flour
- 3 tablespoons. vegetable oil
- ¼ teaspoon pepper
- 1½ pounds round steak
- ½ teaspoon paprika

Directions:

1. Trim excess fat from steak, cut into small pieces. Combine flour, paprika, and pepper and mix. Preheat skillet with oil.
2. Cook steak on both sides. When the color of the steak is brown, remove it to a platter. Add water (150 ml) and stir around the skillet. Return browned steak to skillet; if necessary, add water again so that steak's bottom side does not stick.

Nutrition:
Calories 248
Protein 30 g
Fat 10 g
Carbs 5 g
Phosphorus 190 mg
Potassium 338 mg
Sodium 60 mg

Pork Souvlaki

Preparation time: 20 minutes
Cooking time: 12 minutes
Servings: 8
Ingredients:
- 3 tablespoons olive oil
- 2 tablespoons lemon juice
- 1 teaspoon minced garlic
- 1 tablespoon chopped fresh oregano
- ¼ teaspoon ground black pepper
- 1-pound pork leg, cut into 2-inch cubes

Directions:
1. In a bowl, stir together the lemon juice, olive oil, garlic, oregano, and pepper. Add the pork cubes and toss to coat.
2. Place the bowl in the refrigerator, covered, for 2 hours to marinate. Thread the pork chunks onto 8 wooden skewers that have been soaked in water.
3. Preheat the barbecue to medium-high heat. Grill the pork skewers for about 12 minutes, turning once, until just cooked through but still juicy.

Nutrition:

Calories: 95
Fat: 4g
Carb: 0g
Phosphorus: 125mg
Potassium: 230mg
Sodium: 29mg
Protein: 13g

Ground Chicken & Peas Curry

Preparation Time: 15 minutes
Cooking Time: 6-10 minutes
Servings: 3-4
Ingredients:
- 3 tablespoons essential olive oil
- 2 bay leaves
- 2 onions grind to some paste
- ½ tablespoon garlic paste
- ½ tablespoon ginger paste
- 2 tomatoes, chopped finely
- 1 tablespoon ground cumin
- 1 tablespoon ground coriander
- 1 teaspoon ground turmeric
- 1 teaspoon red chili powder
- Salt, to taste
- 1-pound lean ground chicken
- 2 cups frozen peas
- 1½ cups water
- 1-2 teaspoons garam masala powder

Directions:
1. Warm oil on medium heat in a deep skillet. Add bay leaves and sauté for approximately half a minute. Add onion paste and sauté for about 3-4 minutes.
2. Add garlic and ginger paste and sauté for around 1-1½ minutes. Add tomatoes and spices and cook, occasionally stirring, for about 3-4 minutes.
3. Stir in chicken and cook for about 4-5 minutes. Stir in peas and water and bring to a boil on high heat.
4. Adjust the heat to low and simmer within 5-8 minutes or till the desired doneness. Stir in

garam masala and remove from heat. Serve hot.

Nutrition:
Calories: 450
Fat: 10g
Carbohydrates: 19g
Fiber: 6g
Protein: 38g
Phosphorus 268 mg
Potassium 753.5 mg
Sodium 17 mg

Chicken Meatballs Curry

Preparation Time: 20 min
Cooking Time: 25 minutes

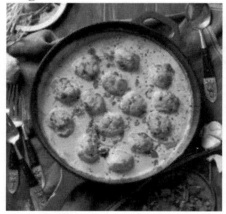

Servings: 3-4
Ingredients:
For Meatballs:
- 1-pound lean ground chicken
- 1 tablespoon onion paste
- 1 teaspoon fresh ginger paste
- 1 teaspoon garlic paste
- 1 green chili, chopped finely
- 1 tablespoon fresh cilantro leaves, chopped
- 1 teaspoon ground coriander
- ½ teaspoon cumin seeds
- ½ teaspoon red chili powder
- ½ teaspoon ground turmeric
- Salt, to taste

For Curry:

- 3 tablespoons extra-virgin olive oil
- ½ teaspoon cumin seeds
- 1 (1-inch) cinnamon stick
- 3 whole cloves
- 3 whole green cardamoms
- 1 whole black cardamom
- 2 onions, chopped
- 1 teaspoon fresh ginger, minced
- 1 teaspoon garlic, minced
- 4 whole tomatoes, chopped finely
- 2 teaspoons ground coriander
- 1 teaspoon garam masala powder
- ½ teaspoon ground nutmeg
- ½ teaspoon red chili powder
- ½ teaspoon ground turmeric
- Salt, to taste
- 1 cup of water
- Chopped fresh cilantro for garnishing

Directions:

1. For meatballs in a substantial bowl, add all ingredients and mix till well combined. Make small equal-sized meatballs from the mixture.
2. Warm-up oil on medium heat in a big deep skillet. Add meatballs and fry approximately 3-5 minutes or till browned from all sides. Transfer the meatballs to a bowl.
3. In the same skillet, add cumin seeds, cinnamon stick, cloves, green cardamom, and black cardamom and sauté for approximately 1 minute.
4. Add onions and sauté for around 4-5 minutes, then put the ginger and garlic paste and sauté within 1 minute. Add tomato and spices and cook, crushing with the spoon's back for about 2-3 minutes.
5. Add water and meatballs and provide to a boil. Reduce heat to low. Simmer for approximately 10 minutes. Serve hot with all the garnishing of cilantro.

Nutrition:
Calories: 421

Fat: 8g
Carbohydrates: 18g
Fiber: 5g
Protein: 34g

Ground Chicken with Basil

Preparation Time: 15 minutes
Cooking Time: 16 minutes
Servings: 8
Ingredients:

- 2 pounds lean ground chicken
- 3 tablespoons coconut oil, divided
- 1 zucchini, chopped
- 1 red bell pepper, seeded and chopped
- ½ of green bell pepper, seeded and chopped
- 4 garlic cloves, minced
- 1 (1-inch) piece fresh ginger, minced
- 1 (1-inch) piece fresh turmeric, minced
- 1 fresh red chili, sliced thinly
- 1 tablespoon organic honey
- 1 tablespoon coconut aminos
- 1½ tablespoons fish sauce
- ½ cup fresh basil, chopped
- Salt
- ground black pepper
- 1 tablespoon fresh lime juice

Directions:

1. Heat a large skillet on medium-high heat. Add ground beef and cook for approximately 5 minutes or till browned completely.
2. Transfer the beef to a bowl. In a similar pan, melt 1 tablespoon of coconut oil on medium-high heat. Add zucchini and bell peppers and stir fry for around 3-4 minutes.
3. Transfer the vegetables inside the bowl with chicken. In precisely the same pan, melt remaining coconut oil on medium heat. Add garlic, ginger, turmeric, and red chili and sauté for approximately 1-2 minutes.
4. Add chicken mixture, honey, and coconut aminos and increase the heat to high. Cook within 4-5 minutes or till sauce is nearly

reduced. Stir in remaining ingredients and take off from the heat.

Nutrition:
Calories: 407
Fat: 7g
Carbohydrates: 20g
Fiber: 13g
Protein: 36g
Phosphorus 149 mg
Potassium 706.3 mg
Sodium 21.3 mg

Chicken &Veggie Casserole

Preparation Time: 15 minutes
Cooking Time: 30 minutes
Servings: 4
Ingredients:

- 1/3 cup Dijon mustard
- 1/3 cup organic honey
- 1 teaspoon dried basil
- ¼ teaspoon ground turmeric
- 1 teaspoon dried basil, crushed
- Salt
- ground black pepper
- 1¾ pound chicken breasts
- 1 cup fresh white mushrooms, sliced
- ½ head broccoli, cut into small florets

Directions:
1. Warm oven to 350 degrees F. Lightly greases a baking dish. In a bowl, mix all ingredients except chicken, mushrooms, and broccoli.
2. Put the chicken in your prepared baking dish, then top with mushroom slices. Place Carrotflorets around chicken evenly.
3. Pour 1 / 2 of honey mixture over chicken and Carrotevenly. Bake for approximately 20 minutes. Now, coat the chicken with the remaining sauce and bake for about 10 minutes.

Nutrition:
Calories: 427

Fat: 9g
Carbohydrates: 16g
Fiber: 7g
Protein: 35g
Phosphorus 353 mg
Potassium 529.3 mg
Sodium 1 mg

Chicken & Cauliflower Rice Casserole

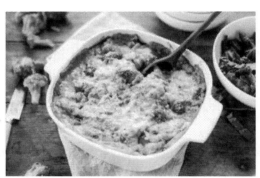

Preparation Time: 15 minutes
Cooking Time: 1 hour & 15 minutes
Servings: 8-10
Ingredients:

- 2 tablespoons coconut oil, divided
- 3-pound bone-in chicken thighs and drumsticks
- Salt
- ground black pepper
- 3 carrots, peeled and sliced
- 1 onion, chopped finely
- 2 garlic cloves, chopped finely
- 2 tablespoons fresh cinnamon, chopped finely
- 2 teaspoons ground cumin
- 1 teaspoon ground coriander
- 12 teaspoon ground cinnamon
- ½ teaspoon ground turmeric
- 1 teaspoon paprika
- ¼ tsp red pepper cayenne
- 1 (28-ounce) can diced tomatoes with liquid
- 1 red bell pepper, thin strips

- ½ cup fresh parsley leaves, minced
- Salt, to taste
- 1 head cauliflower, grated to some rice-like consistency
- 1 lemon, sliced thinly

Directions:
1. Warm oven to 375 degrees F. In a large pan, melt 1 tablespoon of coconut oil at high heat. Add chicken pieces and cook for about 3-5 minutes per side or till golden brown.
2. Transfer the chicken to a plate. In a similar pan, sauté the carrot, onion, garlic, and ginger for about 4-5 minutes on medium heat.
3. Stir in spices and remaining coconut oil. Add chicken, tomatoes, bell pepper, parsley plus salt, and simmer for approximately 3-5 minutes.
4. In the bottom of a 13x9-inch rectangular baking dish, spread the cauliflower rice evenly. Place chicken mixture over cauliflower rice evenly and top with lemon slices.
5. With foil paper, cover the baking dish and bake for approximately 35 minutes. Uncover the baking dish and bake for about 25 minutes.

Nutrition:
Calories: 412
Fat: 12g
Carbohydrates: 23g
Protein: 34g
Phosphorus 201 mg
Potassium 289.4 mg
Sodium 507.4 mg

Chicken Meatloaf with Veggies

Preparation Time: 20 minutes
Cooking Time: 1-1¼ hours
Servings: 4
Ingredients:
For Meatloaf:
- ½ cup cooked chickpeas
- 2 egg whites
- 2½ teaspoons poultry seasoning
- Salt
- ground black pepper
- 10-ounce lean ground chicken
- 1 cup red bell pepper, seeded and minced
- 1 cup celery stalk, minced
- 1/3 cup steel-cut oats
- 1 cup tomato puree, divided
- 2 tablespoons dried onion flakes, crushed
- 1 tablespoon prepared mustard

For Veggies:
- 2-pounds summer squash, sliced
- 16-ounce frozen Brussels sprouts
- 2 tablespoons extra-virgin extra virgin olive oil
- Salt
- ground black pepper

Directions:
1. Warm oven to 350 degrees F. Grease a 9x5-inch loaf pan. In a mixer, add chickpeas, egg whites, poultry seasoning, salt, and black pepper and pulse till smooth.
2. Transfer a combination in a large bowl. Add chicken, veggies oats, ½ cup of tomato puree, and onion flakes and mix till well combined.
3. Transfer the amalgamation into the prepared loaf pan evenly. With both hands, press down the amalgamation slightly.
4. In another bowl, mix mustard and remaining tomato puree. Place the mustard mixture over the loaf pan evenly.
5. Bake approximately 1-1¼ hours or till the desired doneness. Meanwhile, in a big pan of water, arrange a steamer basket. Cover and steam for about 10-12 minutes. Drain well and aside.
6. Now, prepare the Brussels sprouts according to the package's directions. In a big bowl, add veggies, oil, salt, and black pepper and toss to coat well. Serve the meatloaf with veggies.

Nutrition:

Calories: 420
Fat: 9g
Carbohydrates: 21g
Protein: 36g
Phosphorus 237.1 mg
Potassium 583.6 mg
Sodium 136 mg

Roasted Spatchcock Chicken

Preparation Time: 20 minutes
Cooking Time: 50 minutes
Servings: 4-6
Ingredients:

- 1 (4-pound) whole chicken
- 1 (1-inch) piece fresh ginger, sliced
- 4 garlic cloves, chopped
- 1 small bunch of fresh thyme
- Pinch of cayenne
- Salt
- ground black pepper
- ¼ cup fresh lemon juice
- 3 tablespoons extra virgin olive oil

Directions:

1. Arrange chicken, breast side down onto a large cutting board. With a kitchen shear, begin with the thigh, cut along 1 side of the backbone, and turn the chicken around.
2. Now, cut along sleep issues and discard the backbone. Change the inside and open it like a book. Flatten the backbone firmly to flatten.
3. In a food processor, add all ingredients except chicken and pulse till smooth. In a big baking dish, add the marinade mixture.
4. Add chicken and coat with marinade generously. With a plastic wrap, cover the baking dish and refrigerate to marinate overnight.
5. Preheat the oven to 450 degrees F. Arrange a rack in a very roasting pan. Remove the chicken from the refrigerator makes onto a rack over the roasting pan, skin side down.

Roast for about 50 minutes, turning once in a middle way.

Nutrition:
Calories: 419
Fat: 14g
Carbohydrates: 28g
Protein: 40g
Phosphorus 166 mg
Potassium 196 mg
Sodium 68 mg

Roasted Chicken with Veggies & Orange

Preparation Time: 20 minutes
Cooking Time: 1 hour
Servings: 4
Ingredients:

- 1 teaspoon ground ginger
- ½ teaspoon ground cumin
- ½ teaspoon ground coriander
- 1 teaspoon paprika
- Salt
- ground black pepper
- 1 (3 ½-4-pound) whole chicken
- 1 unpeeled orange, cut into 8 wedges
- 2 medium carrots, peeled and cut 1nto 2-inch pieces
- 2 medium sweet potatoes, peeled and cut into ½-inch wedges
- ½ cup of water

Directions:

1. Warm oven to 450 degrees F. In a little bowl, mix the spices. Rub the chicken with spice mixture evenly.
2. Arrange the chicken in a substantial Dutch oven and put the orange, carrot, and sweet potato pieces around it.
3. Add water and cover the pan tightly. Roast for around 30 minutes. Uncover and roast for about half an hour.

Nutrition:
Calories: 432

Fat: 10g
Carbohydrates: 20g
Protein: 34g
Potassium 481 mg
Sodium 418 mg
Phosphorus 170 mg

Roasted Chicken Breast

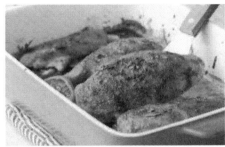

Preparation Time: 15 minutes
Cooking Time: 40 minutes
Servings: 4-6
Ingredients:

- ½ of a small apple, peeled, cored, and chopped
- 1 bunch scallion, trimmed and chopped roughly
- 8 fresh ginger slices, chopped
- 2 garlic cloves, chopped
- 3 tablespoons essential olive oil
- 12 teaspoon sesame oil, toasted
- 3 tablespoons using apple cider vinegar
- 1 tablespoon fish sauce
- 1 tablespoon coconut aminos
- Salt
- ground black pepper
- 4-pounds chicken thighs

Directions:

1. Pulse all the fixing except chicken thighs in a blender. Transfer a combination and chicken right into a large Ziploc bag and seal it.
2. Shake the bag to marinade well. Refrigerate to marinate for about 12 hours. Warm oven to 400 degrees F. Arranges a rack in foil paper-lined baking sheet.
3. Place the chicken thighs on the rack, skin-side down. Roast for about 40 minutes, flipping once within the middle way.

Nutrition:
Calories: 451
Fat: 17g
Carbohydrates: 277g
Protein: 42g
Phosphorus 121 mg
Potassium 324 mg
Sodium 482.9 mg

PICO DE GALLO

Servings: 12 | Prep: 20m | Cooks: 3h20m | Total:3hm | Additional: 3h

INGREDIENTS

6 roma (plum) tomatoes, diced
1 clove garlic, minced
1/2 red onion, minced
1 pinch garlic powder
3 tablespoons chopped fresh cilantro
1 pinch ground cumin, or to taste
1/2 jalapeno pepper, seeded and minced
salt and ground black pepper to taste
1/2 lime, juiced

DIRECTIONS

1 the tomatoes, onion, cilantro, jalapeno pepper, lime juice,garlic, garlic powder, cumin, salt, and pepper together in a bowl.
2. Refrigerate at least 3 hours before serving.

NUTRITION FACTS
Calories: 10 | Carbohydrates: 2.2g | Fat: 0.1g | Protein: 0.4g |Cholesterol: 0m

Grilled Chicken

Preparation Time: 15 minutes
Cooking Time: 41 minutes
Servings: 8
Ingredients:

- 1 (3-inch) piece fresh ginger, minced
- 6 small garlic cloves, minced
- 1½ tablespoons tamarind paste
- 1 tablespoon organic honey
- ¼ cup coconut aminos
- 2½ tablespoons extra virgin olive oil
- 1½ tablespoons sesame oil, toasted
- ½ teaspoon ground cardamom
- Salt
- ground white pepper
- 1 (4-5-pound) whole chicken, cut into 8 pieces

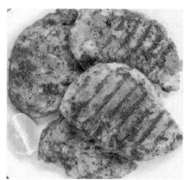

Directions:
1. Mix all ingredients except chicken pieces in a large glass bowl. With a fork, pierce the chicken pieces thoroughly.
2. Add chicken pieces in bowl and coat with marinade generously. Cover and refrigerate to marinate for approximately a couple of hours to overnight.
3. Preheat the grill to medium heat. Grease the grill grate. Place the chicken pieces on the grill, bone-side down. Grill, covered approximately 20-25 minutes.
4. Change the side and grill, covered approximately 6-8 minutes. Change alongside it and grill, covered for about 5-8 minutes. Serve.

Nutrition:
Calories: 423
Fat: 12g
Carbohydrates: 20g

Protein: 42g
Sodium 281.9 mg
Phosphorus 0 mg
Potassium 0 mg

Grilled Chicken with Pineapple & Veggies

Preparation Time: 20 or so minutes
Cooking Time: 22 minutes
Servings: 4
Ingredients:
For Sauce:
- 1 garlic oil, minced
- ¾ teaspoon fresh ginger, minced
- ½ cup coconut aminos
- ¼ cup fresh pineapple juice
- 2 tablespoons freshly squeezed lemon juice
- 2 tablespoons balsamic vinegar
- ¼ teaspoon red pepper flakes, crushed
- Salt
- ground black pepper

For Grilling:
- 4 skinless, boneless chicken breasts
- 1 pineapple, peeled and sliced
- 1 bell pepper, seeded and cubed
- 1 zucchini, sliced
- 1red onion, sliced

Directions:
1. For sauce in a pan, mix all ingredients on medium-high heat. Bring to a boil reducing the heat to medium-low. Cook approximately 5-6 minutes.
2. Remove, then keep aside to cool down slightly. Coat the chicken breasts about ¼ from the sauce. Keep aside for approximately half an hour.
3. Preheat the grill to medium-high heat. Grease the grill grate. Grill the chicken pieces for around 5-8 minutes per side.
4. Now, squeeze pineapple and vegetables on the grill grate. Grill the pineapple within 3 minutes per side. Grill the vegetables for

approximately 4-5 minutes, stirring once inside the middle way.

5. Cut the chicken breasts into desired size slices, divide the chicken, pineapple, and vegetables into serving plates. Serve alongside the remaining sauce.

Nutrition:
Calories: 435
Fat: 12g
Carbohydrates: 25g
Protein: 38g
Phosphorus 184 mg
Potassium 334.4 mg
Sodium 755.6 mg

Ground Turkey with Veggies

Preparation Time: 15 minutes
Cooking Time: 12 minutes
Servings: 4
Ingredients:
- 1 tablespoon sesame oil
- 1 tablespoon coconut oil
- 1-pound lean ground turkey
- 2 tablespoons fresh ginger, minced
- 2 minced garlic cloves
- 1 (16-ounce) bag vegetable mix (broccoli, carrot, cabbage, kale, and Brussels sprouts)
- ¼ cup coconut aminos
- 2 tablespoons balsamic vinegar

Directions:
1. In a big skillet, heat both oils on medium-high heat. Add turkey, ginger, and garlic and cook approximately 5-6 minutes. Add vegetable mix and cook about 4-5 minutes. Stir in coconut aminos and vinegar and cook for about 1 minute. Serve hot.

Nutrition:
Calories: 234
Fat: 9g
Carbohydrates: 9g
Protein: 29g

Phosphorus 14 mg
Potassium 92.2 mg
Sodium 114.9 mg

Ground Turkey with Asparagus

Preparation Time: 15 minutes
Cooking Time: 15 minutes
Servings: 8
Ingredients:
- 1¾ pound lean ground turkey
- 2 tablespoons sesame oil
- 1 medium onion, chopped
- 1 cup celery, chopped
- 6 garlic cloves, minced
- 2 cups asparagus, cut into 1-inch pieces
- 1/3 cup coconut aminos
- 2½ teaspoons ginger powder
- 2 tablespoons organic coconut crystals
- 1 tablespoon arrowroot starch
- 1 tablespoon cold water
- ¼ teaspoon red pepper flakes, crushed

Directions:
1. Heat a substantial nonstick skillet on medium-high heat. Add turkey and cook for approximately 5-7 minutes or till browned. With a slotted spoon, transfer the turkey inside a bowl and discard the grease from the skillet.
2. Heat-up oil on medium heat in the same skillet. Add onion, celery, and garlic and sauté for about 5 minutes. Add asparagus and cooked turkey, minimizing the temperature to medium-low.
3. Meanwhile, inside a pan, mix coconut aminos, ginger powder, and coconut crystals n medium heat and convey some boil.
4. Mix arrowroot starch and water in a smaller bowl. Slowly add arrowroot mixture, stirring continuously. Cook approximately 2-3 minutes.
5. Add the sauce in the skillet with turkey mixture and stir to blend. Stir in red pepper

flakes and cook for approximately 2-3 minutes. Serve hot.

Nutrition:
Calories: 309
Fat: 20g
Carbohydrates: 19g
Protein: 28g
Potassium 196.4 mg
Sodium 77.8 mg
Phosphorus 0 mg

Ground Turkey with Peas & Potato

Preparation Time: 15 minutes
Cooking Time: 35 minutes
Servings: 4
Ingredients:

- 3-4 tablespoons coconut oil
- 1-pound lean ground turkey
- 1-2 fresh red chilis, chopped
- 1 onion, chopped
- Salt, to taste
- 2 minced garlic cloves
- 1 (1-inch) piece fresh ginger, grated finely
- 1 tablespoon curry powder
- 1 teaspoon ground coriander
- 1 teaspoon ground cumin
- 1 teaspoon ground turmeric
- 2 large Yukon gold potatoes, cubed into 1-inch size
- ½ cup of water
- 1 cup fresh peas, shelled
- 2-4 plum tomatoes, chopped
- ½ cup fresh cilantro, chopped

Directions:
1. In a substantial pan, heat oil on medium-high heat. Add turkey and cook for about 4-5 minutes. Add chilis and onion and cook for about 4-5 minutes.
2. Add garlic and ginger and cook approximately 1-2 minutes. Stir in spices, potatoes, and water and convey to your boil

3. Reduce the warmth to medium-low. Simmer covered around 15-20 or so minutes. Add peas and tomatoes and cook for about 2-3 minutes. Serve using the garnishing of cilantro.

Nutrition:
Calories: 452
Fat: 14g
Carbohydrates: 24g
Fiber: 13g
Protein: 36g
Phosphorus 38 mg
Potassium 99.5 mg
Sodium 373.4 mg

Turkey & Pumpkin Chili

Preparation Time: 15 minutes
Cooking Time: 41 minutes
Servings: 4-6
Ingredients:

- 2 tablespoons extra-virgin olive oil
- 1 green bell pepper, seeded and chopped
- 1 small yellow onion, chopped
- 2 garlic cloves, chopped finely
- 1-pound lean ground turkey
- 1 (15-ounce) pumpkin puree
- 1 (14 ½-ounce) can diced tomatoes with liquid
- 1 teaspoon ground cumin
- ½ teaspoon ground turmeric
- ½ teaspoon ground cinnamon
- 1 cup of water
- 1 can chickpeas, rinsed and drained

Directions:
1. Heat-up oil on medium-low heat in a big pan. Add the bell pepper, onion, and garlic and sauté for approximately 5 minutes. Add turkey and cook for about 5-6 minutes.
2. Add tomatoes, pumpkin, spices, and water and convey to your boil on high heat. Reduce the temperature to medium-low heat and stir in chickpeas. Simmer, covered for

approximately a half-hour, stirring occasionally. Serve hot.

Nutrition:
Calories: 437
Fat: 17g
Carbohydrates: 29g
Protein: 42g
Phosphorus 150 mg
Potassium 652 mg
Sodium 570 mg

Chicken Kebab Sandwich

Preparation time: 15 minutes
Cooking time: 15 minutes
Servings: 4
Ingredients:

- 12 ounces boneless, skinless chicken breast
- 2 tablespoons freshly squeezed lemon juice
- 1 tablespoon extra-virgin olive oil
- 4 garlic cloves, minced, divided
- Freshly ground black pepper
- ¼ cup plain, unsweetened yogurt
- 4 white flatbreads
- 1 cucumber, sliced
- 1 cup lettuce, shredded

Directions:
1. In a medium bowl, add the chicken breast, lemon juice, olive oil, and half the garlic, tossing to coat. Season with pepper. Set aside to marinate.
2. Put the yogurt and remaining garlic in a small bowl. Season with pepper and mix well. Set aside. Heat-up a large skillet over medium-high heat, and add the chicken and the marinade.
3. Cook for 5 minutes. Flip, then cook until the chicken is golden brown and the juices run clear.
4. Remove from the pan and let rest for 5 minutes. Cut the chicken into thin slices. In each flatbread, add some chicken, cucumber,

and lettuce. Top with the yogurt sauce, and serve.

Nutrition:
Calories: 217
Fat: 6g
Carbohydrates: 21g
Protein: 22g
Phosphorus: 80mg
Potassium: 231mg
Sodium: 339mg

Aromatic Chicken and Cabbage Stir-Fry

Preparation time: 10 minutes

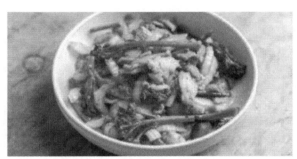

Cooking time: 10 minutes
Servings: 4
Ingredients:

- 1 teaspoon canola oil
- 10 ounces boneless, skinless chicken breast, thinly sliced
- 3 cups green cabbage, thinly sliced
- 1 tablespoon cornstarch
- 1 teaspoon ground ginger
- ½ teaspoon garlic powder
- ¼ cup of water
- Freshly ground black pepper

Directions:
1. Heat-up the oil in a large skillet over medium-high heat. Add the chicken and cook, often stirring, until browned and cooked through. Put the cabbage in the pan, then cook for another 2 to 3 minutes.

2. Mix the cornstarch, ginger, garlic, and water in a small bowl. Add the mixture to the pan, and continue cooking until the sauce has slightly thickened about 1 minute. Season with pepper.

Nutrition:
Calories: 96
Fat: 2g
Carbohydrates: 5g
Protein: 15g
Phosphorus: 15mg
Potassium: 140mg
Sodium: 156mg

Chicken Chow Mein

Preparation time: 10 minutes
Cooking time: 15 minutes
Servings: 6
Ingredients:
- 2 teaspoons cornstarch
- 1 tablespoon water
- 1 teaspoon low-sodium soy sauce
- 1 teaspoon of rice wine
- 1 teaspoon sugar
- 1 teaspoon sesame oil
- 2 teaspoons canola oil
- 3 garlic cloves, minced
- 8 oz chicken thighs, thinly sliced
- 2 cups shredded green cabbage
- 1 carrot, julienned
- 4 scallions, cut into 2-inch pieces
- 10 oz chow Mein noodles, cooked
- 1 cup mung bean sprouts

Directions:
1. Mix the cornstarch, water, plus soy sauce in a small bowl. Stir in the rice wine, sugar, plus sesame oil, then set aside. Heat-up the canola oil in a large skillet or wok over medium-high heat.
2. Put the garlic, and cook until just fragrant. Put the chicken, and cook within 1 minute, stirring, until the chicken is browned but not cooked. Add the cabbage, carrot, and scallions, cook for 1-2 minutes.
3. Put the noodles, and toss with the chicken and vegetables. Put in the sauce, and mix to coat, then put the bean sprouts, and stir. Remove from the heat, and serve.

Nutrition:
Calories: 342
Fat: 18g
Carbohydrates: 34g
Protein: 13g
Phosphorus: 169mg
Potassium: 308mg
Sodium: 289mg

Baked Herbed Chicken

Preparation time: 10 minutes
Cooking time: 40 minutes
Servings: 6
Ingredients:
- 4 tablespoons Fat free butter or coconut spread, at room temperature
- 4 garlic cloves, minced
- 1 tablespoon chopped fresh oregano
- 1 tablespoon chopped fresh parsley
- 1 teaspoon lemon zest
- 6 bone-in chicken thighs
- ¼ teaspoon freshly ground black pepper

Directions:
1. Preheat the oven to 425°F. Mix the Fat free butter or coconut spread, garlic, oregano, parsley, and lemon zest in a small bowl.
2. Arrange the thighs on a baking tray and gently peel back the skin, leaving it attached. Brush the thigh meat with a couple of teaspoons of the Fat free butter or coconut spread mixture, and replace the skin to cover the meat. Season with pepper.
3. Bake within 40 minutes, until the skin is crisp and the juices run clear. Let rest for 5 minutes before serving.

Nutrition:
Calories: 226
Fat: 17g
Carbohydrates: 1g
Protein: 16g
Phosphorus: 114mg
Potassium: 158mg
Sodium: 120mg

Chicken Satay with Peanut Sauce

Preparation time: 10 minutes
Cooking time: 10 minutes
Servings: 6
Ingredients:
For the Chicken:

- ½ cup plain, unsweetened yogurt
- 2 garlic cloves, minced
- 1-inch piece ginger, minced
- 2 teaspoons curry powder
- 1-pound chicken breast, boneless, skinless, cut into strips
- 1 teaspoon canola oil

For the Peanut Sauce:

- ¾ cup smooth unsalted peanut Fat free butter or coconut spread
- 1 teaspoon soy sauce
- 1 tablespoon brown sugar
- Juice of 2 limes
- ½ teaspoon red chili flakes
- ¼ cup hot water
- Fresh cilantro leaves, chopped, for garnish
- Lime wedges, for garnish

Directions:
1. In a small bowl, add the yogurt, garlic, ginger, and curry powder. Stir to mix. Add the chicken strips to the marinade. Cover and refrigerate for 2 hours.
2. Thread the chicken pieces onto skewers. Oiled a grill pan using the canola oil and heat on medium-high. Cook the chicken skewers on each side for 3 to 5 minutes, until cooked through.
3. Mix the peanut Fat free butter or coconut spread, soy sauce, brown sugar, lime juice, red chili flakes, and hot water in a food processor. Process until smooth.
4. Transfer then sprinkle with the cilantro. Serve with the chicken satay along with lime wedges for squeezing over the skewers.

Nutrition:
Calories: 286
Fat: 18g
Carbohydrates: 10g
Protein: 25g
Phosphorus: 33mg
Potassium: 66mg
Sodium: 201mg

Oven Baked Chicken Teriyaki

Servings: 4 | Prep: 15m | Cooks: 35m | Total: 50m

INGREDIENTS
2 tablespoons cornstarch
4 teaspoons grated fresh ginger
2 tablespoons water
3 cloves garlic, minced
1 cup low-sodium soy sauce
1/4 teaspoon red pepper flakes
1/2 cup stevia
4 skinless, boneless chicken breast halves

DIRECTIONS
Preheat oven to 400 degrees F (200 degrees C). Whisk cornstarch and water together in a small bowl until dissolved; set aside. Combine soy sauce, stevia, ginger, garlic,and red pepper flakes together in a saucepan over medium heat untilthe mixture starts to simmer. Slowly whisk in cornstarch mixture. Bring to a boil; reduce heat to mediumlow, and simmer until thickened, stirring often, about 10 minutes.

Pat chicken dry with paper towels; arrange in a baking dish. Poursauce over chicken breasts, coating all sides.

Bake chicken breasts in the preheated oven until no longer pink inthe center and the juices run clear, 25 to 30 minutes. An instant-read thermometer inserted into the center should read at least 165 degrees F (75 degrees C).

NUTRITION FACTS

Calories: 315 | Carbohydrates: 39.9g | Fat: 2.9g | Protein: 28.1g |Cholesterol: 67mg

Zucchini Cookies

Servings: 36 | Prep: 15m | Cooks: 10m | Total:25m

INGREDIENTS

1/2 cup margarine, softened
1 teaspoon baking soda
1 cup white sugar
1/2 teaspoon salt
1 egg
1 teaspoon ground cinnamon
1 cup grated zucchini
1/2 teaspoon ground cloves
2 cups all-purpose flour
1 cup raisins

DIRECTIONS

In a medium bowl, cream together the margarine and sugar until smooth. Beat in the egg then stir in the zucchini. Combine the flour, baking soda, salt and cinnamon; stir into the zucchini mixture. Mix inraisins. Cover dough and chill for at least 1 hour or overnight.

Preheat oven to 375 degrees F (190 degrees C). Grease cookie sheets. Drop dough by teaspoonfuls onto the prepared cookie sheet. Cookies should be about 2 inches apart.

Bake for 8 to 10 minutes in the preheated oven until set. Allow cookies to cool slightly on the cookie sheets before removing to wireracks to cool completely.

NUTRITION FACTS

Calories: 81 | Carbohydrates: 13.4g | Fat: 2.7g | Protein: 1 g |Cholesterol: 5mg

Vegetarian and Vegan Entrees

SPICED SWEET ROASTED RED PEPPER HUMMUS

Servings: 4 |
Prep: 15m
Cooks: 10m
Total: 25m

INGREDIENTS

1 (15 ounce) can garbanzo beans, drained
1/2 teaspoon ground cumin
1 (4 ounce) jar roasted red peppers
1/2 teaspoon cayenne pepper
3 tablespoons lemon juice
1/4 teaspoon salt
1 1/2 tablespoons tahini
1 tablespoon chopped fresh parsley
1 garlic minced

DIRECTIONS

In an electric blender or food processor, puree the chickpeas, redpeppers, lemon juice, tahini, garlic, cumin, cayenne, and salt. Process, using long pulses, until the mixture is fairly smooth, and slightly fluffy. Make sure to scrape the mixture off the sides of the food processor or blender in between pulses. Transfer to a serving bowl and refrigerate for at least 1 hour. (The hummus can be madeup to 3 days ahead and refrigerated. Return to room temperature before serving.)
Sprinkle the hummus with the chopped parsley before serving.

NUTRITION FACTS

Calories: 64 | Carbohydrates: 9.6g |
Fat: 2.2g | Protein: 2.5g |
Cholesterol: 0mg

LENTIS VEGAN SOUP

Preparation Time: 10 minutes

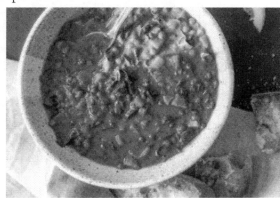

Cooking Time: 50 minutes
Servings: 5
Ingredients

- 2 tablespoons olive oil
- 1 onion, diced
- 2 cloves garlic, minced
- 1 carrot, chopped
- 2 potatoes, diced
- 1 can of tomato, diced
- 2 cups dried lentil
- 8 cups vegetable broth
- 1 bay leaf
- 1/2 tsp cumin
- salt, as per taste
- pepper, as per taste

Directions:
1. Start by taking a large pot and add in 2 tablespoons of olive oil. Place the pot over medium flame.
2. Once the oil heats through, toss in the onions and cook for 5 minutes. Put in the garlic and cook gain within 2 minutes.
3. Now toss in the diced potatoes and carrots. Sauté for about 3 minutes. Add the remaining ingredients like vegetable broth, tomatoes, lentils, cumin, and bay leaf.

4. Once boiling, adjust to low and cook for about 40 minutes. Discard the bay leaf and season with pepper and salt. Transfer into a serving bowl. Serve hot!

Nutrition
Calories: 364
Fat: 7g
Carbohydrates: 58g
Protein: 19g
Potassium 0 mg
Sodium 287.1 mg
Phosphorus 0mg

Carrot Casserole

Preparation Time: 15 minutes

Cooking Time: 15 minutes

Servings: 4

Ingredients

- ½ pound carrots
- ½ cup graham crackers
- 1 tablespoon olive oil
- 1 tablespoon onion
- 1/8 teaspoon black pepper
- 1/6 cup shredded cheddar cheese
- Salt

Directions:
1. Preheat oven to 350° F.
2. Slice the peeled carrots into 1/4-inch rounds. Put the carrots in a large saucepan over medium-high heat and boil. Drain and set aside 1/3-cup liquid.
3. Mash carrots until they are smooth. Crush graham crackers, heat oil, and minced onion. Place in a greased small casserole dish. Serve hot.

Nutrition
Calories: 118
Carbs: 16g
Fat: 8g
Protein: 3g
Sodium: 86mg
Potassium: 205mg
Phosphorus: 189mg

Chinese Tempeh Stir Fry

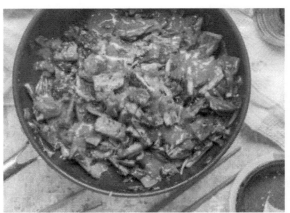

Preparation time: 5 minutes

Cooking time: 15 minutes

Servings: 2

Ingredients:

- 2 oz. sliced tempeh
- 1 cup cooked brown rice
- 1 minced garlic clove
- ½ cup green onions
- 1 tsp minced fresh ginger
- 1 tbsp coconut oil
- ½ cup of corn

Direction:
1. Heat-up the oil in a skillet or wok on high heat and add the garlic and ginger. Sauté for 1 minute. Now add the tempeh and cook for 5-6 minutes before adding the corn for a further 10 minutes. Now add the green onions and serve over brown rice.

Nutrition
Calories: 304
Protein: 10g
Carbs: 35g
Fat: 4g
Sodium: 91mg
Potassium: 121mg
Phosphorus: 222mg

Green Velvet Soup

Servings: 8 | Prep: 10m | Cooks: 1h20m | Total:1h30m

INGREDIENTS:
- 1 onion, chopped
- 2 zucchini, diced
- 2 stalks celery, sliced
- 1 head broccoli, chopped
- 2 potatoes, diced
- 1/2 teaspoon dried basil
- 3/4 cup dried split peas
- 1/4 teaspoon ground black pepper
- 2 bay leaves
- 4 cups chopped fresh spinach
- 6 cups vegetable broth
- salt to taste

DIRECTIONS

In a large pot over medium heat, combine onion, celery, potatoes,split peas, bay leaves and broth. Bring to a boil, then reduce heat, cover and simmer 1 hour.
Remove the bay leaves and stir in the zucchini, broccoli, basil andblack pepper. Simmer 20 minutes, until broccoli is tender.
Stir in spinach and remove from heat. Puree in a blender or foodprocessor using an immersion blender. Salt to taste.
NUTRITION
Calories: 120
Carbohydrates: 24.4g|
Fat: 0.8g
Protein: 5.5g
Cholesterol: 0mg □

Carrot with Garlic Fat free butter or coconut spread and Almonds

Preparation Time: 10 minutes
Cooking Time: 50 minutes
Servings: 3
Ingredients:

- 1-pound fresh broccoli, cut into bite-size pieces
- ¼ cup olive oil
- ½ tablespoon honey
- 1-1/2 tablespoons soy sauce
- ¼ teaspoon ground black pepper
- 2 cloves garlic, minced
- ¼ cup chopped almonds

Directions:
1. Cook the Carrotinto a large pot with 1-inch of water in the bottom. Drain, and arrange Carroton a serving platter. Heat-up oil in a small skillet over medium heat. Mix in the honey, soy sauce, pepper, and garlic.
2. Boil, then remove from the heat. Mix in the almonds, and pour the sauce over the broccoli. Serve immediately.

Nutrition
Calories: 177
Sodium: 234mg
Protein: 2.9g
Carbs: 2g
Fat: 2g
Potassium: 13mg
Phosphorus: 67mg

Hearty Vegan Slow Cooker Chilli

Servings: 15 | Prep: 45m | Cooks: 5h10m | Total:5h55m
INGREDIENTS
1 tablespoon olive oil
1 tablespoon dried oregano
1 green bell pepper, chopped
1 tablespoon dried parsley
1 red bell pepper, chopped
1/2 teaspoon salt
1 yellow bell pepper, chopped
1/2 teaspoon ground black pepper
2 onions, chopped
2 (14.5 ounce) cans diced tomatoes with juice
4 cloves garlic, minced
1 (15 ounce) can black beans, rinsed and drained

1 (10 ounce) package frozen chopped spinach, thawed anddrained
1 (15 ounce) can garbanzo beans, drained
1 cup frozen corn kernels, thawed
1 (15 ounce) can kidney beans, rinsed and drained
1 zucchini, chopped
2 (6 ounce) cans tomato paste
1 yellow squash, chopped
1 (8 ounce) can tomato sauce, or more if needed
6 tablespoons chili powder
1 cup vegetable broth, or more if needed
1 tablespoon ground cumin

DIRECTIONS

Heat olive oil in a large skillet over medium heat, and cook the green, red, and yellow bell peppers, onions, and garlic until the onions start to brown, 8 to 10 minutes. Place the mixture into a slow cooker. Stir in spinach, corn, zucchini, yellow squash, chili powder, cumin, oregano, parsley, salt, black pepper, tomatoes, black beans, garbanzo beans, kidney beans, and tomato paste until thoroughly mixed. Pour the tomato sauce and vegetable broth over the ingredients.

Set the cooker on Low, and cook until all vegetables are tender, 4to 5 hours. Check seasoning; if chili is too thick, add more tomato sauce and vegetable broth to desired thickness. Cook an additional 1 to 2 hours to blend the flavors.

NUTRITION FACTS
Calories: 134 | Carbohydrates: 24.8g | Fat: 2.4g | Protein: 6.3g |Cholesterol: 0mg

Thai Tofu Broth

Preparation time: 5 minutes
Cooking time: 15 minutes
Servings: 4
Ingredients:
- 1 cup of rice noodles
- ½ sliced onion
- 6 oz. drained, pressed, and cubed tofu
- ¼ cup sliced scallions
- ½ cup of water
- ½ cup canned water chestnuts
- ½ cup of rice milk
- 1 tbsp lime juice
- 1 tbsp coconut oil
- ½ finely sliced chili
- 1 cup snow peas

Directions:
1. Heat-up the oil in a wok on high heat and then sauté the tofu until brown on each side. Add the onion and sauté for 2-3 minutes. Add the rice milk and water to the wok until bubbling.
2. Lower to medium heat and add the noodles, chili, and water chestnuts. Allow to simmer for 10-15 minutes, and then add the stevia or aspartame snap peas for 5 minutes. Serve with a sprinkle of scallions.

Nutrition
Calories: 304
Protein: 9g
Carbs: 38g
Fat: 13g
Sodium: 36mg
Potassium: 114mg
Phosphorus: 101mg

Broccoli Steaks

Preparation Time: 10 minutes
Cooking Time: 25 minutes
Servings: 2
Ingredients:
- 1 medium head Broccoli
- 3 tablespoons unsalted Fat free butter or coconut spread
- ¼ teaspoon garlic powder
- ¼ teaspoon onion powder
- 1/8 teaspoon salt
- ¼ teaspoon pepper

Directions:

1. Preheat the oven to 400 degrees F. Please parchment paper on a roasting pan.
2. Trim the leaves off the broccoli and cut off the bottom of the stem. Cut the broccoli head in half. Cut each half into 1 to 3/4-inch slices, leaving the core in place.
3. Cut off the smaller ends of the broccoli and save for another recipe. There should be 4 broccoli steaks. Mix Fat free butter or coconut spread, garlic powder, onion powder, salt, and pepper.
4. Lay the broccoli on the parchment-lined baking sheet. Using half of the Fat free butter or coconut spread mixture, brush onto the steaks. Put in the preheated oven within 20 minutes.
5. Remove, then flip the steaks over. Brush steaks with the rest of the Fat free butter or coconut spread and roast for about 20 more minutes, until they are golden brown on the edges.

Nutrition:
Calories: 86
Sodium: 143mg
Protein: 0.8g
Carbs: 2g
Fat: 13g
Potassium: 80mg
Phosphorus: 61mg

Roasted Garlic Lemon Cauliflower

Preparation Time: 10 minutes
Cooking Time: 15 minutes
Servings: 4
Ingredients:
- 2 heads cauliflower, separated into florets
- 2 teaspoons olive oil
- ½ teaspoon ground black pepper
- 1 clove garlic, minced
- ½ teaspoon lemon juice

Directions:

1. Warm oven to 400 degrees F. Bake in the preheated oven within 15 to 20 minutes. Transfer to a serving platter, then serve.

Nutrition:
Calories: 37
Sodium: 27mg
Protein: 1.8g
Carbs: 15g
Fat: 10g
Potassium: 272mg
Phosphorus: 161mg

Carrot with Garlic Sauce

Preparation Time: 10 minutes
Cooking Time: 15 minutes
Servings: 3
Ingredients:
- 2 cups Carrot florets
- 1 garlic clove
- ½ tablespoon Fat free butter or coconut spread
- 2 teaspoons honey
- 1-1/2 tablespoons apple cider vinegar
- 1 tablespoon fresh parsley

Directions:
1. Steam Carrotover boiling water within 8 to 10 minutes in a large saucepan with a steamer rack. Mix in the honey, apple cider vinegar plus chopped parsley. Put the saucepan to heat until sauce is heated. Transfer steamed Carrotto a serving dish. Pour sauce over hot Carrotand toss to coat.

Nutrition
Calories: 41
Sodium: 26mg
Protein: 1.4g
Carbs: 22g
Fat: 8g
Potassium: 157mg
Phosphorus: 100 mg

Zesty Zucchini And Squash

Servings: 6 | Prep: 15m | Cooks: 25m | Total: 40m

INGREDIENTS

3 medium small yellow squash, cubed

1/2 onion, chopped

3 small zucchini, cubed

salt to taste

1 (10 ounce) can diced tomatoes with green chile peppers

garlic powder to taste

In a large saucepan, combine squash, zucchini, tomatoes withchiles, onion, salt and garlic powder. Bring to a boil over medium-high heat. Reduce heat to low and cook until tender-crisp.

NUTRITION FACTS

Calories: 43 | Carbohydrates: 9.7g | Fat: 0.4g | Protein: 1.8g |Cholesterol: 0mg

Parsley Root Veg Stew

Preparation time: 5 minutes

Cooking time: 35-40 minutes

Servings: 4

Ingredients:

- 2 garlic cloves
- 2 cups white rice
- 1 tsp ground cumin
- 1 diced onion
- 2 cups of water
- 4 peeled and diced turnips
- 1 tsp cayenne pepper
- ¼ cup chopped fresh parsley
- ½ tsp ground cinnamon
- 2 tbsp olive oil
- 1 tsp ground ginger
- 2 peeled and diced carrots

Directions:

1. Heat-up oil on medium-high heat in a large pot before sautéing the onion for 4-5 minutes

until soft. Put the turnips and cook within 10 minutes or until golden brown.

2. Add the garlic, cumin, ginger, cinnamon, and cayenne pepper, cooking for a further 3 minutes. Add the carrots and stock to the pot, and then bring to the boil.

3. Turn the heat down to medium heat, cover, and simmer for 20 minutes. Meanwhile, add the rice to a pot of water and bring to a boil.

4. Turn down to simmer for 15 minutes. Drain and place the lid on for 5 minutes to steam. Garnish the root vegetable stew with parsley to serve alongside the rice.

Nutrition:

Calories: 210

Protein: 4g

Carbs: 32g

Fat: 7g

Sodium: 67mg

Potassium: 181mg

Phosphorus: 105mg

Sautéed Green Beans

Preparation Time: 10 minutes

Cooking Time: 15 minutes

Servings: 5

Ingredients:

- 2 cup frozen green beans
- ½ cup red bell pepper
- 4 tsp margarine
- ¼ cup onion
- 1 tsp dried dill weed
- 1 tsp dried parsley
- ¼ tsp black pepper

Directions:

1. Cook green beans in a large pan of boiling water until tender, then drain. While the beans are cooking, melt the margarine in a skillet and fry the other vegetables.

2. Add the beans to sautéed vegetables. Sprinkle with freshly ground pepper and serve with meat and fish dishes.

Nutrition:
Calories: 67
Carbs: 8g
Protein: 4g
Fat: 5g
Potassium: 192mg
Phosphorous: 32mg
Sodium: 458 mg

Couscous with Vegetables

Preparation Time: 10 minutes
Cooking Time: 15 minutes
Servings: 5
Ingredients:

- 1 tbsp margarine
- ½ cup frozen peas
- ½ cup onion, minced
- ¼ cup mushrooms, sliced
- ½ cup couscous, uncooked
- 1 garlic clove, minced
- 2 tbsp dry white wine
- ½ tsp dried basil
- ¼ tsp black pepper
- 1 tbsp dried parsley

Directions:
1. Dissolve the margarine in a skillet over medium-high heat. Sauté the peas, onion, mushrooms, garlic, and wine. Add the herbs.
2. Prepare the couscous according to package instructions. Toss the vegetables through the hot couscous and serve.

Nutrition:
Calories 104
Carbs: 18g
Protein: 3g
Fat: 2g
Potassium: 100g
Phosphorous: 52mg
Sodium: 160 mg

Grill Thyme Corn on the Cob

Preparation Time: 10 minutes
Cooking Time: 20 minutes
Servings: 3
Ingredients:

- 1 tbsp grated Parmesan cheese
- 4 half-ear size corn on the cob, frozen
- ½ tsp dried thyme
- ¼ tsp black pepper
- 2 tbsp olive oil

Directions:
1. In a small bowl, mix the oil, cheese, thyme, and black pepper. Coat the corn in the oil mixture. Place the corn in a foil packet topped with 2 ice cubes. Place the corn on a grill and cook for approximately 20 minutes.

Nutrition:
Calories: 125
Carbs: 11g
Protein: 4g
Fat: 7g
Potassium: 164g
Phosphorous: 57mg
Sodium: 14 mg

Ginger Glazed Carrots

Preparation Time: 10 minutes
Cooking Time: 20 minutes
Servings: 3
Ingredients:

- 2 cups carrots, sliced into 1-inch pieces
- ¼ cup apple juice
- 2 tbsp margarine, melted
- ¼ cup boiling water
- 1 tbsp. stevia or aspartame
- 1 tsp cornstarch
- ¼ tsp salt
- ¼ tsp ground ginger

Directions:

1. Cook carrots until tender. Mix sugar, cornstarch, salt, ginger, apple juice, and margarine together 3. Pour mixture over carrots and cook for 10 minutes until thickened. Serve.

Nutrition:
Calories: 101
Carbs: 14g
Protein: 1g
Fat: 2g
Potassium: 202g
Phosphorous: 26mg
Sodium: 65g

Spring Vegetables with Tofu

Preparation time: 15 minutes
Cooking time: 10 minutes
Servings: 4
Ingredients:
- 500 g green asparagus
- alternatively: 2 yellow or red peppers
- 1 bunch of spring onions
- 350 g pointed cabbage
- 1 bowl of watercress
- 1 package (100 g) mixed sprouts
- 25 g fresh ginger
- 2 cloves of garlic
- 1 dried chili pepper
- 3-4 tbsp soy sauce
- 3 tbsp lime juice
- 4 tbsp oil
- 300 g tofu
- to turn: whole meal spelled flour

Directions:
1. Slice off the asparagus' woody ends, slice the stalks into pieces about 2 cm wide. Wash, core, and, alternatively, cut the peppers into suitable pieces.
2. Slice the spring onions into pieces. It cleans and washes pointed cabbage, cutting out the stalk. Cut fine cabbage strips. Clean, dry, spin,

and rinse. Plug them into bits bite-sized. Peel and chop ginger and garlic. Dried chili crumbles. Combine in a bowl soy sauce and lime juice. Add the sesame oil.
3. Heat a wok or deep pan with 2 tablespoons of oil. Cut the tofu into bite-sized pieces and mix with some whole meal flour. Fry in hot oil until brown. Season with salt and pepper. Use kitchen paper to remove/drain. Drain that oil.
4. Heat the remaining wok oil. Fry asparagus for 1-2 minutes while stirring. Fry onions and cabbage and the remaining vegetables for a minute. Combine marinade, fold pieces of tofu. Season with salt and pepper. Serve.

Nutrition:
Calories 383
Fat 24 g
Carbohydrates 20 g
Protein 22 g
Potassium 170 mg
Sodium 140 mg
Phosphorous: 0mg

Asparagus and Carrot Salad with Burrata

Preparation time: 15 minutes
Cooking time: 8 minutes
Servings: 2
Ingredients:
- 250 g white asparagus
- 250 g green asparagus
- 2 carrots
- 3 tbsp olive oil
- 1 tbsp sunflower seeds
- 1 tbsp lemon juice
- 150 g cherry tomatoes
- 1 handful arugula
- 1 spring onion
- 2 bullets burrata

Directions:
1. Peel the asparagus, and the lower ends are cut off. Wash the green asparagus, and the woody

ends are also cut off. Cut it into pieces with the asparagus. Clean, peel, and cut into sticks with the carrots.

2. In a saucepan, heat the oil and fry the asparagus and carrots over medium heat for 5 minutes. Add the seeds to the sunflower and roast for 3 minutes.
3. Deglaze with lemon juice and add salt and pepper to season the asparagus and carrot mix. Take it off the stove then and let it cool down.
4. Wash the tomatoes and quarter them at the same time. Rocket wash and dry shake. The spring onions are cleaned, washed, and cut into pieces.
5. Mix the tomatoes, rocket, and spring onions with the asparagus, arrange them on plates and serve each with a scoop of burrata.

Nutrition:
Calories 671
Protein 34 g
Fat 48 g
Carbohydrates 26 g
Phosphorus 31 mg
Potassium 286.6 mg

Quinoa Salad

Preparation time: 15 minutes
Cooking time: 10 minutes
Servings: 4
Ingredients:

- 200 g quinoa
- 1 mango
- 1 cucumber
- 3 tomatoes
- 1 red pepper
- 150 g lamb's lettuce
- 1 red onion
- 2 stems mint
- 150 g feta (45% fat in dry matter)
- 1 tbsp olive oil
- 1 tbsp apple cider vinegar
- salt

- pepper

Directions:

1. Rinse the quinoa with cold water, bring to the boil in a saucepan with twice the amount of water and cook over low heat for about 10 minutes.
2. In the meantime, peel the mango, cut from the stone, and dice the pulp. Clean, wash, and cut the cucumber, tomatoes, and peppers. Wash the lamb's lettuce and spin dry. Peel and chop the onion. Wash the mint, shake dry, pluck the leaves and cut into strips. Dice the feta.
3. Drain the quinoa, drain and transfer to a bowl. Add the mango, cucumber, tomatoes, bell pepper, lamb's lettuce, onion, mint, feta, and mix. Season the salad with olive oil, apple cider vinegar, salt, and pepper. Serve.

Nutrition:
Calories 409
Protein 15 g
Fat 16 g
Carbohydrates 50 g
Phosphorus 347 mg
Potassium 321.3 mg
Sodium 331.9 mg

Spinach Mango Vegetables

Preparation time: 15 minutes
Cooking time: 10 minutes
Servings: 2
Ingredients:

- 750 g young spinach leaves
- 2 bunch spring onions, cut into pieces about 2 cm wide
- 2 ripe mangos, cut it into cubes about 1 cm in size
- 2 tbsp germ oil
- 1 ginger
- 2 tbsp sunflower seeds
- 20 g amaranth pops
- salt

- cayenne pepper

Directions:
1. Heat-up 1 tablespoon of oil in a saucepan and cook the covered spring onions over medium heat for about 5 minutes. Put the spinach and cook within 5 minutes, covered.
2. Meanwhile, peel the ginger and finely grate it, collecting the juice. Add the spinach to the mango cubes, ginger and ginger juice, and cover and heat for about 3 minutes over medium heat.
3. Meanwhile, in a coated pan, heat the remaining oil. Roast the sunflower seeds for 3-4 minutes over low heat, then add the pops of amaranth.
4. Season the salted spinach and mango vegetables and arrange them on a plate. Sprinkle over the vegetables and season the roasted sunflower seeds, and amaranth pops with cayenne pepper.

Nutrition:
Calories 240
Protein 8 g
Fat 10 g
Carbohydrates 27 g
Phosphorus 883 mg
Potassium 1 mg
Sodium 146.1 mg

Braised Swiss Chard

Preparation time: 15 minutes
Cooking time: 10 minutes
Servings: 2
Ingredients:
- 1 large bunch of Swiss chard
- 1 tbsp. olive oil
- 2 cloves of garlic, minced
- 1/4 tsp. red pepper flakes
- 1 tbsp balsamic vinegar or lemon juice

Directions:
1. Clean the leaves and cut their base. Add oil and garlic to a preheated skillet. Add the

chilies and leaves, then stir over high heat until the leaves are tender. Add vinegar or lemon juice. Serve with crushed pepper.

Nutrition:
Calories: 88
Protein: 1.4 g
Carbohydrates: 5.4 g
Fat: 7 g
Sodium: 165 mg
Phosphorus: 42 mg
Potassium: 314 mg

Snow Peas All with Thyme

Preparation time: 15 minutes
Cooking time: 6 minutes
Servings: 4
Ingredients:
- 2 tbsp margarine
- 2 tbsp fresh lemon juice
- Zest of one lemon
- 1 tsp dried thyme
- ½ pound snow peas, trimmed

Directions:
1. Melt the margarine in a shallow pot. Combine lemon zest and juice, and thyme set aside. Steam the snow peas for 3 minutes over boiling water or in the microwave on high for 3 minutes until tender. Drain and fold into the mixture. Serve.

Nutrition:
Calories: 45 g
Proteins: 2 g
Carbohydrates: 5 g
Fat: 2.4 g
Sodium: 30 mg
Phosphorus: 42.6 mg
Potassium: 296 mg

Cauliflower and Fresh Dill

Preparation time: 15 minutes
Cooking time: 10 minutes

Servings: 2
Ingredients:
- 1 medium cauliflower head, cut into florets
- 2 tbsp. lemon juice
- 1 tbsp. olive oil
- 1/3 cup fresh dill, chopped
- Pepper to taste

Directions:
1. Cook the florets within 10 minutes in a large pot of boiling water, covered; drain out the cauliflower. Transfer to a dish for serving.
2. Mix the oil plus the lemon juice; pour the cauliflower over it and mix. Sprinkle with dill and sprinkle with pepper to taste. Serve.

Nutrition:
Calories: 45 g
Proteins: 2 g
Carbohydrates: 5 g
Fat: 2.4 g
Sodium: 30 mg
Phosphorus: 42.6 mg
Potassium: 296 mg

Zucchini and Corn Stir-Fry

Preparation time: 5 minutes
Cooking time: 10 minutes
Servings: 2
Ingredients:
- 2 medium zucchinis, diced
- 2 cups frozen corn
- 1 medium red pepper, diced
- 1 tbsp chili flakes
- 1 tbsp vegetable oil

Directions:
1. Heat the oil in a pan. Add vegetables and chili, cook over high heat until zucchini is tender. Serve.

Nutrition:
Calories: 67 g
Proteins: 2 g

Carbohydrates: 11 g
Fat: 2 g
Sodium: 6 mg
Phosphorus: 53 mg
Potassium: 253 mg

Marinated Zucchini

Preparation time: 15 minutes
Cooking time: 0 minutes
Servings: 1-8
Ingredients:
- 500 g zucchini
- 30 g extra virgin olive oil
- 4 tablespoons of lemon juice
- 4 tablespoons of apple (or rice) cider vinegar
- 2 cloves of garlic
- 2 sprigs of mint
- 1 dry chili
- 1 pinch of salt

Directions:
2. Wash the zucchini well, check the two ends, and cut them into skinny slices lengthwise using a mandolin or a potato peeler. Wash the mint and dry it, remove a few leaves that you will keep whole, and chop the rest of the leaves.
3. For the marinade, mix the lemon with the vinegar and oil in a bowl, add the chopped mint, salt, and crumbled red pepper.
4. In a rectangular container of suitable length, arrange the zucchini slices lined up in layers and season with the marinade, alternating between the layers a few pieces of garlic and a few whole mint leaves.
5. Let it rest in the fridge within 5 hours. Remove from the refrigerator 10 minutes before serving.

Nutrition:
Calories: 81
Protein: 2 g
Carbs 8.53 g
Fat 27.5 g

Phosphorus 30.1 mg
Potassium 233.1 mg
Sodium 517.8 mg

"Cooked Water"

Preparation time: 15 minutes
Cooking time: 60 minutes
Servings: 4
Ingredients:

- 400 g potatoes
- 300 g field chicory
- 200 g artichokes
- 100 g onion
- 100 g ripe tomatoes
- 100 g onion
- chili
- mint
- 200 g unsalted bread
- 40 g extra virgin olive oil

Directions:
1. Put the peeled and halved potatoes; put the halved artichokes, 3-4 whole garlic cloves, sliced onions, mint, chili pepper, and chopped tomatoes in a saucepan only water and salt.
2. Cook for about 1 hour. When cooked, add one egg per person, poached in the broth of the same soup.
3. During cooking, you have to pay attention to keep a certain amount of liquid by adding hot water. When cooked, pour the broth on the bread, making sure you have all the ingredients for each dish.
4. Let it rest for a few minutes with the plate covered. The bread can get wet properly, then throw away the liquid not absorbed by the bread and sprinkle the soup abundantly with extra virgin olive oil.

Nutrition:
Calories: 429
Protein: 17 g
Fat 1.8 g

Phosphorous: 306 mg
Potassium: 1296 mg
Carbs: 54 g
Sodium: 209 mg

Tofu Stir Fry

Preparation time: 15 minutes

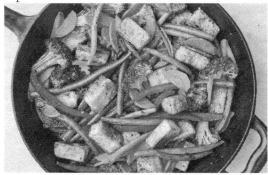

Cooking time: 20 minutes
Servings: 4
Ingredients:

- 1 teaspoon stevia or aspartame
- 1 tablespoon lime juice
- 1 tablespoon low-sodium soy sauce
- 2 tablespoons cornstarch
- 2 egg whites, beaten
- 1/2 cup unseasoned bread crumbs
- 1 tablespoon vegetable oil
- 16 ounces tofu, cubed
- 1 clove garlic, minced
- 1 tablespoon sesame oil
- 1 red bell pepper, sliced into strips
- 1 cup Carrotflorets
- 1 teaspoon herb seasoning blend
- Dash black pepper
- Sesame seeds
- Steamed white rice.

Directions:
1. Dissolve stevia or aspartamein a mixture of lime juice and soy sauce. Set aside. In the first bowl, put the cornstarch. Add the egg whites to the second bowl. Place the breadcrumbs in the third bowl.

2. Dip each tofu cubes in the first, second, and third bowls. Pour vegetable oil into a pan over medium heat, then cook tofu cubes until golden.
3. Drain the tofu and set aside. Remove the oil from the pan and add sesame oil, then put garlic, bell pepper, and broccoli. Cook until crisp-tender. Season with the seasoning blend and pepper.
4. Put the tofu back and toss to mix. Pour soy sauce mixture on top and transfer to serving bowls. Garnish with the sesame seeds and serve on top of white rice.

Nutrition:
Calories: 401
Carbs: 0g
Protein: 19g
Fats: 0g
Sodium: 584mg
Potassium: 317mg
Phosphorus: 177mg

Carrot Pancake

Preparation time: 10 minutes
Cooking time: 25 minutes
Servings: 4
Ingredients:
- 3 cups carrot , diced
- 2 tablespoons all-purpose flour
- 1/2 cup onion, chopped
- 2 tablespoons olive oil.

Directions:
1. Cut and Boil the carrots in water for 15/20 minutes.
2. When ready , mashed and Add onion, flour and olive oil to the mixture. And mix
3. Create the pancake shape and cook it until is brown on both sides. Serve.

Nutrition:
Calories: 140
Protein: 6 g
Fats: 0g

Carbs: 0g
Sodium: 58mg
Potassium: 276mg
Phosphorus: 101mg.

Grilled Squash

Preparation time: 10 minutes
Cooking time: 6 minutes
Servings: 8
Ingredients:
- 4 zucchinis, rinsed, drained, and sliced
- 4 crookneck squash, rinsed, drained, and sliced
- Cooking spray
- 1/4 teaspoon garlic powder
- 1/4 teaspoon black pepper.

Directions:
1. Arrange squash on a baking sheet. Spray with oil. Season with garlic powder and pepper. Grill within 3 minutes per side or until tender but not too soft. Serve.

Nutrition:
Calories: 17
Protein: 1g
Potassium: 262mg
Phosphorus: 39mg
Carbs: 0g
Fats: 0g

Vegetarian Lasagna

Preparation time: 10 minutes
Cooking time: 1 hour
Servings: 4
Ingredients:
- 1 teaspoon basil
- 1 tablespoon olive oil
- ½ sliced red pepper
- 3 egg free lasagna sheets
- ½ diced red onion
- ¼ teaspoon black pepper
- 1 cup of rice milk

- 1 minced garlic clove
- 1 cup sliced eggplant
- ½ sliced zucchini
- ½ pack soft tofu
- 1 teaspoon oregano.

Directions:
1. Preheat oven to 325°F. Slice zucchini, eggplant, and pepper into vertical strips. Add the rice milk and tofu to a food processor and blitz until smooth. Set aside.
2. Heat-up oil in a skillet over medium heat and add the onions and garlic for 3-4 minutes or until soft. Sprinkle in the herbs and pepper and allow to stir through for 5-6 minutes until hot.
3. Into a lasagna or suitable oven dish, layer 1 lasagna sheet, then 1/3 the eggplant, followed by 1/3 zucchini, then 1/3 pepper before pouring over 1/3 of white tofu sauce.
4. Repeat for the next 2 layers, finishing with the white sauce. Add to the oven for 40-50 minutes or until veg is soft and easily be sliced into servings.

Nutrition:
Calories: 235
Protein: 5 g
Carbs: 10g
Fat: 9 g
Sodium: 35mg
Potassium: 129mg
Phosphorus: 66mg

Chili Tofu Noodles

Preparation time: 5 minutes
Cooking time: 15 minutes
Servings: 4
Ingredients:
- ½ diced red chili
- 2 cups of rice noodles
- ½ juiced lime
- 6 ounces pressed and cubed silken firm tofu
- 1 teaspoon grated fresh ginger

- 1 tablespoon coconut oil
- 1 cup green beans
- 1 minced garlic clove.

Directions:
1. Steam the green beans for 10-12 minutes or according to package directions and drain. Cook the noodles in a pot of boiling water for 10-15 minutes or according to package directions.
2. Meanwhile, warm a wok or skillet on high heat and add coconut oil. Now add the tofu, chili flakes, garlic, and ginger and sauté for 5-10 minutes.
3. After doing that, drain the noodles and the green beans and lime juice and then add it to the wok. Toss to coat. Serve hot!

Nutrition:
Calories: 246
Protein: 10g
Carbs: 28g
Fat: 12 g
Sodium: 25mg
Potassium: 126mg
Phosphorus: 79mg.

Curried Cauliflower

Preparation time: 5 minutes
Cooking time: 20 minutes
Servings: 4
Ingredients:
- 1 teaspoon turmeric
- 1 diced onion
- 1 tablespoon chopped fresh cilantro
- 1 teaspoon cumin
- ½ diced chili
- ½ cup of water
- 1 minced garlic clove
- 1 tablespoon coconut oil
- 1 teaspoon gram masala
- 2 cups cauliflower florets.

Directions:

1. Warm-up oil in a skillet on medium heat. Sauté the onion and garlic for 5 minutes until soft. Add in the cumin, turmeric, and gram masala and stir to release the aromas.
2. Now add the chili to the pan along with the cauliflower. Stir to coat. Pour in the water and reduce the heat to a simmer for 15 minutes. Garnish with cilantro to serve.

Nutrition:
Calories: 108
Protein: 2g
Carbs: 11g
Fat: 7g
Sodium: 35mg
Potassium: 328mg
Phosphorus: 39mg.

Elegant Veggie Tortillas

Preparation time: 30 minutes
Cooking time: 15 minutes
Servings: 12
Ingredients:
- 1½ cups of chopped Carrotflorets
- 1½ cups of chopped cauliflower florets
- 1 tablespoon of water
- 2 teaspoon of canola oil
- 1½ cups of chopped onion
- 1 minced garlic clove
- 2 tablespoons of finely chopped fresh parsley
- 1 cup of low-cholesterol liquid egg substitute
- Freshly ground black pepper, to taste
- 4 (6-ounce) warmed corn tortillas.

Directions:
1. In a microwaveable bowl, place broccoli, cauliflower, and water and microwave, covered for about 3-5 minutes. Remove, then drain any liquid.
2. Heat oil on medium heat. Add onion and sauté for about 4-5 minutes. Add garlic and then sauté it for about 1 minute, then stir in the broccoli, cauliflower, parsley, egg substitute, and black pepper.

3. Reduce the heat and it to simmer for about 10 minutes. Remove then set aside to cool slightly. Place Carrotmixture over ¼ of each tortilla.
4. Fold the outside edges inward and roll up like a burrito. Secure each tortilla with toothpicks to secure the filling. Cut each tortilla in half and serve.

Nutrition:
Calories: 217
Fat: 3.3g
Carbs: 41g
Protein: 8.1g
Phosphorus: 0g
Potassium: 289mg
Sodium: 87mg

Sweet and Sour Chickpeas

Preparation time: 10 minutes
Cooking time: 12 minutes
Servings: 6
Ingredients:
- 2 tablespoons extra-virgin olive oil
- 1 onion, chopped
- 1 (14-ounce) can tropical fruit in fruit juice, strained, reserving juice
- 2 tablespoons freshly squeezed lemon juice
- 2 tablespoons cornstarch
- 2 (15-ounce) cans no-salt-added chickpeas, drained and rinsed.

Directions:
1. Heat-up olive oil over medium heat in a large saucepan. Cook the onion within 4 to 5 minutes, frequently stirring, until tender.
2. Mix the fruit juice, lemon juice, and cornstarch in a medium bowl. When the onion is tender, add the chickpeas and cook for 3 to 4 minutes, stirring until hot.
3. Add the juice mixture and cook, frequently stirring, until the liquid is thickened, about 2 minutes. Add the drained fruits to the saucepan and simmer for 1 to 2 minutes or until hot. Serve.

Nutrition:
Calories: 333
Sodium: 15mg
Phosphorus: 253mg
Potassium: 505mg
Fats: 0g
Carbs: 0g
Protein: 13g

Cabbage-Stuffed Mushrooms

Preparation time: 20 minutes
Cooking time: 25 minutes
Servings: 6
Ingredients:

- 6 Portobello mushrooms
- 3 tablespoons extra-virgin olive oil
- 1 onion, chopped
- 1 teaspoon minced peeled fresh ginger
- 2 cups shredded red cabbage
- 1/8 teaspoon salt
- 1/8 teaspoon freshly ground black pepper
- 3 tablespoons water
- 1 cup shredded Monterey Jack cheese.

Directions:

1. Rinse the mushrooms briefly and pat dry. Remove the stems, then discard. Scrape out the dark gills on the mushroom cap using a spoon. Set aside.
2. Heat-up the olive oil over medium heat in a medium skillet and cook the onion and ginger for 2 to 3 minutes, stirring until it is fragrant.
3. Add the cabbage, salt, and pepper and sauté for 3 minutes, stirring frequently. Add the water, cover, and steam the cabbage for 3 to 4 minutes, or until it is tender.
4. Remove the vegetables, then put in a medium bowl; let cool for 10 minutes, then stir in the cheese. Preheat the oven to 400°F.
5. Put the caps on a baking sheet and divide the filling among the mushrooms. Bake for 15 to 17 minutes, or until the mushrooms are tender and the filling is light golden brown. Serve.

Nutrition:
Calories: 163
Sodium: 179mg
Phosphorus: 173mg
Potassium: 360mg
Fats: 0g
Carbs: 0g
Protein: 7g.

Curried Veggie Stir-Fry

Preparation time: 20 minutes
Cooking time: 10 minutes
Servings: 6
Ingredients:

- 2 tablespoons extra-virgin olive oil
- 1 onion, chopped
- 4 garlic cloves, minced
- 4 cups frozen stir-fry vegetables
- 1 cup canned unsweetened full-fat coconut milk
- 1 cup of water
- 2 tablespoons green curry paste.

Directions:

1. Heat-up the olive oil over medium-high heat in a wok or nonstick skillet. Stir-fry the onion and garlic for 2 to 3 minutes, until fragrant.
2. Add the frozen stir-fry vegetables and continue to cook for 3 to 4 minutes longer, or until the vegetables are hot.
3. Meanwhile, in a small bowl, combine coconut milk, water, and curry paste. Stir until the paste dissolves.
4. Put the broth batter to the wok and cook for another 2 to 3 minutes. Serve over couscous or hot cooked rice.

Nutrition:
Calories: 293
Sodium: 247mg
Phosphorus: 138mg
Potassium: 531mg
Fats: 0g
Carbs: 0g

Protein: 7g

Creamy Mushroom Pasta

Preparation time: 10 minutes
Cooking time: 20 minutes
Servings: 6
Ingredients:

- 12 ounces whole-grain fettuccine pasta
- 3 tablespoons extra-virgin olive oil
- 1 (8-ounce) package button mushrooms, sliced
- 3 garlic cloves, sliced
- 1 cup heavy cream
- pinch salt
- freshly ground black pepper.

Directions:

1. Boil a pot of water, then cook the pasta within 9 to 10 minutes, until al dente. Drain, then set aside about 1/3 cup of the pasta water and set aside.
2. Meanwhile, in a large, heavy saucepan, heat the olive oil on medium-high heat. Add the mushrooms in a single layer. Cook for 3 minutes or until the mushrooms are golden brown on one side.
3. Carefully turn the mushrooms and cook for another 2 minutes. Adjust the heat to medium, then put the garlic. Sauté, stirring, for 2 minutes longer, until the garlic is fragrant.
4. Put the cream in the skillet with the mushrooms and season with salt and pepper. Simmer within 3 minutes or until the mixture starts to thicken.
5. Put your drained pasta in the pan and coat using tongs. Add the reserved pasta water if necessary to loosen the sauce. Serve.

Nutrition:
Calories: 405
Sodium: 42mg
Phosphorus: 252mg
Potassium: 410mg

Fats: 0g
Carbohydrates: 44g
Protein: 10g

CarrotStir-Fry

Preparation time: 40 minutes
Cooking time: 15 minutes
Servings: 4
Ingredients:

- 1 tablespoon of olive oil
- 1 minced garlic clove
- 2 cups of Carrotflorets
- 2 tablespoons of water.

Directions:

1. Heat oil on medium heat. Add garlic and then sauté for about 1 minute. Put the Carrotand stir fry within 2 minutes. Stir in water and stir fry for about 4-5 minutes. Serve warm.

Nutrition:
Calories: 47
Fat: 3.6g
Carbs: 3.3g
Protein: 1.3g
Phosphorus: 0g
Potassium: 147mg
Sodium: 15mg

Salad with Strawberries and Goat Cheese

Preparation time: 15 minutes
Cooking time: 0 minute
Servings: 2
Ingredients:

- Baby lettuce, to taste
- 1-pint strawberries
- Balsamic vinegar
- Extra virgin olive oil
- 1/4 teaspoon black pepper
- 8-ounce soft goat cheese.

Directions:

1. Prepare the lettuce by washing and drying it, then cut the strawberries. Cut the soft goat cheese into 8 pieces. Put together the balsamic vinegar and the extra virgin olive oil in a large cup with a whisk.
2. Mix the strawberries pressing them and putting them in a bowl, add the dressing and mix, divide the lettuce into four dishes, and cut the other strawberries, arranging them on the salad. Put cheese slices on top and add pepper. Serve and enjoy!

Nutrition:
Calories: 300
Protein: 13g
Fat: 0g
Carbs: 0g
Sodium: 285mg
Potassium: 400mg
Phosphorus: 193mg

Winter Spiced Squash Stew

Preparation time: 15 minutes
Cooking time: 6 hours
Servings: 6
Ingredients:
- 1 spaghetti squash
- 2 medium zucchinis
- 1/2 cup of yellow bell pepper
- 1 cup of unsweetened canned pineapple, diced
- ½ cup of water
- 1 tsp of allspice
- 2 ½ tbsp of brown stevia or aspartame
- 1 tbsp of unsalted Fat free butter or coconut spread

Directions:
1. Cut the squashes down the middle (horizontally). Dice the bell pepper into small pieces. Placed the squash halves into the slow cooker (skin side up).
2. In a small bowl, mix the pepper, pineapple, ½ cup of water, allspice, brown sugar, and melted Fat free butter or coconut spread. Pour the mix into the slow cooker around the base of the squash.
3. Cover the squash and cook on a Low for 6-7 hours or until squash is tender. Stir the pot gently to mix the ingredients well before serving.

Nutrition:
Calories: 63
Protein: 1g
Carbohydrates: 10g
Fat: 3g
Sodium: 18mg
Potassium: 309mg
Phosphorus: 37mg

Vegetable Stew with Mediterranean Spices

Preparation time: 15 minutes
Cooking time: 1 hour
Servings: 4
Ingredients:
- 1 zucchini, sliced
- 2 red bell peppers, sliced
- 2 eggplants, diced
- 2 medium white onions, diced
- 3 cups of water
- 1 cup of low sodium vegetable stock (optional)
- 1 tsp of dried thyme
- 1 tsp of nutmeg
- 1 tsp of paprika
- 1 tbsp of cider vinegar
- 1 tbsp of ground black pepper
- 1 tbsp all-purpose flour
- 2 garlic cloves, peeled and halved
- 2 cups white rice
- 2 tbsp fresh basil, chopped

Directions:
1. Roughly chop the vegetables into large pieces. Boil the water in a saucepan. Mix the flour with the boiled water until the lumps dissolve.

2. Now add all the fixing into the slow cooker. Cook on low within 1-2 hours or until the vegetables are soft and the sauce is thickened. Serve with fluffy white rice and a garnish of fresh basil.

Nutrition:
Calories: 154
Protein: 4g
Carbohydrates: 34g
Fat: 1g
Sodium: 132mg
Potassium: 380mg
Phosphorus: 85mg

Root Vegetable Roast

Preparation time: 15 minutes
Cooking time: 3 hours
Servings: 6
Ingredients:
- 1 rutabaga, peeled and cubed
- 2 large carrots, peeled and cubed
- 2 turnips, peeled and cubed
- 2 cups of water
- 1 tbsp of all-purpose flour
- 1 garlic clove, minced
- 1 cup of low sodium vegetable stock (optional)
- 2 tbsp dried oregano
- 1 tbsp black pepper
- 1 loaf of crusty white bread

Directions:
1. Peel and chop the rutabaga, carrots, and turnips into cubes. Boil the water and stir in the flour until lumps have dissolved.
2. Add all of the remaining ingredients to the slow cooker. Cook on a low 3-4 hours or until vegetables is tender. Serve in hearty bowls.

Nutrition:
Calories: 144
Protein: 5g

Carbohydrates: 29g
Fat: 1g
Sodium: 265mg
Potassium: 388mg
Phosphorus: 92mg

Soft Red Cabbage with Cranberry

Preparation time: 15 minutes
Cooking time: 1 hour
Servings: 5
Ingredients:
- 2 red cabbages
- 1 cup of canned cranberries, juices drained
- 1 tsp of balsamic vinegar
- 1 tsp of allspice
- 1 tsp of ground black pepper
- 1 tsp of brown stevia or aspartame
- 2 cups of water

Directions:
1. Wash and slice the red cabbage, making sure it's not too thin. Throw all of the fixings into the slow cooker. Cook on low within 1 hour or until the cabbage is soft. Enjoy this as a main dish with rice or noodles or as a side dish.

Nutrition:
Calories: 107
Protein: 2g
Carbohydrates: 27g
Fat: 0g
Sodium: 50mg
Potassium: 335mg
Phosphorus: 44mg

Cabbage with Cucumber and Dill Relish

Preparation time: 15 minutes
Cooking time: 1 hour & 30 minutes
Servings: 4
Ingredients:
- 1 white cabbage
- 1 tbsp. of olive oil

- 1 lemon, juice squeezed
- A pinch of black pepper
- 1 cucumber, diced
- 1 tbsp of fresh or dried dill

Directions:
1. Slice the cabbage into strips. Dissolve the Fat free butter or coconut spread over medium heat in a skillet and add the juice from half the lemon (save one half for serving).
2. Pour this into the slow cooker and add in the cabbage. Cover with a little water just to reach the top of the cabbage.
3. Cook on a Low with the lid on for 1 ½ hour. Remove the cover and continue to cook if it's still a bit watery for 10 minutes.
4. Prepare your salad by dicing the cucumber and mixing it in the dill. Squeeze the leftover lemon juice into the salad. Serve a helping of the cabbage with the cold cucumber relish.

Nutrition:
Calories: 73
Protein: 2g
Carbohydrates: 10g
Fat: 4g
Sodium: 13mg
Potassium: 375mg
Phosphorus: 61mg

Coconut & Pecan Sweet Potatoes

Preparation time: 20 minutes
Cooking time: 4-5 hours
Servings: 16
Ingredients:
- 4 lb. sweet potatoes, peeled and diced
- ½ cup pecans, chopped
- ½ cup unsweetened flaked coconut
- ½ cup Fat free butter or coconut spread, melted
- 1/3 cup sugar
- 1/3 cup brown stevia or aspartame
- ½ tsp vanilla extract
- ¼ tsp low sodium salt

Directions:
1. Place the sweet potatoes in a 5 quart or larger slow cooker. Mix the pecans, coconut, melted

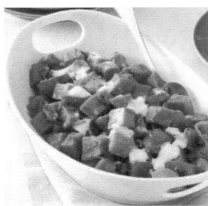

Fat free butter or coconut spread, both sugars, vanilla extract, and salt. Toss the nut mixture with the sweet potatoes. Cover and cook on low for 4 to 5 hours. Serve.

Nutrition:
Calories 307
Fat 16g
Carbs 42g
Protein 3g
Phosphorus: 0g
Potassium 419mg
Sodium 50mg

Veggie Bolognese

Preparation time: 20 minutes
Cooking time: 8-10 hours
Servings: 32
Ingredients:
- 1 onion, diced
- 7 medium carrots, peeled & diced
- 2 green bell peppers, diced
- 3 small zucchinis, diced
- 2 cups mushrooms, roughly chopped
- 87oz canned crushed tomatoes
- 2 tbsp dried basil
- 1 tbsp dried oregano
- 1 tsp dried rosemary

- 1 whole bay leaf, crumbled
- 3 garlic cloves, minced

Directions:
1. Place all ingredients into a 6-quart or larger slow cooker and mix well. Cover and cook on LOW within 8 to 10 hours. Serve.

Nutrition:
Calories 43
Fat >1g
Carbs 10g
Protein 2g
Potassium 411mg
Sodium 112mg
Phosphorus 3 mg

Bombay Potatoes

Preparation time: 45 minutes
Cooking time: 4-6 hours
Servings: 6
Ingredients:
- 3 tbsp olive oil
- 2 tsp mustard seeds
- 1 onion, peeled and diced
- 1 teaspoon Garam Masala Spice
- 1 tsp ground ginger
- 1 ½ tsp turmeric
- ½ tsp ground cumin
- ½ tsp chili powder
- ¼ tsp red chili flakes
- 3 lb. potatoes, peeled and diced into ½ inch cubes
- 14.5oz canned low-sodium diced tomatoes or fresh tomatoes
- 1 tsp low sodium salt
- ½ tsp freshly ground black pepper
- ¼ cup fresh cilantro, finely chopped

Directions:
1. Cook the mustard seeds in a large skillet until they begin to pop. Add the onions are spices and cook for a further 5 minutes.

2. Add the potatoes, tomatoes, and onion mixture to a 6-quart slow cooker and cover. Cook within 4 to 6 hours on low.

Nutrition:
Calories 280
Fat 8g
Carbs 10g
Protein 2g
Potassium 911mg
Sodium 78mg
Phosphorus 149 mg

Potato & CarrotGratin

Preparation time: 20 minutes
Cooking time: 3-4 hours
Servings: 6
Ingredients:
- 5 medium potatoes, sliced
- 2 cup Carrotflorets, chopped
- ½ tsp freshly ground black pepper
- ½ tsp low sodium salt
- ¼ cup unsalted margarine
- ¼ cup all-purpose flour
- 1 medium onion, minced
- 1 garlic clove, minced
- 1 cup milk
- 1 cup low-sodium Cheddar cheese

Directions:
1. Arrange the potato slices and Carrotflorets in a 4 to 6-quart slow cooker. Dissolve the margarine in a saucepan and put the flour to make a roux.
2. Gradually whisk in the milk, then add the garlic, onion, and cheese. Pour the sauce over potatoes and cover. Cover and cook on high within 3 to 4 hours.

Nutrition:
Calories 444
Fat 21g
Carbs 49g
Protein 2g

Potassium 1106mg
Sodium 378mg

Summer Squash with Bell Pepper and Pineapple

Preparation time: 15 minutes
Cooking time: 6-7 hours
Serves 6
Ingredients:

- 1 lb. summer squash, peeled and cubed
- 1 lb. zucchini squash, peeled and cubed
- ½ cup green bell pepper, chopped
- 1 8oz can unsweetened crushed pineapple
- 1 tsp ground cinnamon
- 1/3 cup brown stevia or aspartame
- 1 tbsp Fat free butter or coconut spread, cut into small pieces

Directions:
1. Mix all fixing and place in a 4 to 6-quart slow cooker. Cover and cook on low for 6-7 hours or until squash is tender. Serve immediately.

Nutrition:
Calories 113
Fat 2g
Carbs 24g
Protein 2g
Potassium 381mg
Sodium 7mg
Phosphorus: 0g

Soup and Stews

Low-Sodium Chicken Broth

Preparation Time: 10 minutes
Cooking Time: 4 minutes
Servings: 8
Ingredients:

- 2 pounds skinless whole chicken, cut into pieces
- 4 garlic cloves, lightly crushed
- 2 celery stalks, with greens, roughly chopped
- 2 carrots, roughly chopped
- 1 sweet onion, cut into quarters
- 10 peppercorns
- 4 fresh thyme sprigs
- 2 bay leaves
- Water

Directions:

1. In a large stockpot, place the chicken, garlic, celery, carrots, onion, peppercorns, thyme, and bay leaves, and cover with water about 3 inches.
2. Boil the water over high heat, then adjust the heat to medium-low and simmer, uncovered, for about 4 hours. Remove any foam on top of the stock, and pour the stock through a fine-mesh sieve.
3. Pick off all the usable chicken meat for another recipe, discard the bones and other solids, and allow the stock to cool for about 30 minutes before transferring it to sealable containers.

Nutrition:
Calories: 32
Fat: 0 g
Sodium: 57 mg
Carbs: 8 g
Protein: 1 g
Potassium: 0 mg
Phosphorous: 0 mg

Turkey Soup

Servings: 12 | Prep: 45m | Cooks: 2h | Total: 2h45m
INGREDIENTS
1 turkey carcass
1 tablespoon Worcestershire sauce
4 quarts water
1 1/2 teaspoons salt
6 small potatoes, diced
1 teaspoon dried parsley
4 large carrots, diced
1 teaspoon dried basil
2 stalks celery, diced
1 bay leaf
1 large onion, diced
1/4 teaspoon freshly cracked black pepper
1 1/2 cups shredded cabbage
1/4 teaspoon paprika
1 (28 ounce) can whole peeled tomatoes, chopped
1/4 teaspoon poultry seasoning
1/2 cup uncooked barley
1 pinch dried thyme
DIRECTIONS

1. Place the turkey carcass into a large soup pot or stock pot and pour in the water; bring to a boil, reduce heat to a simmer, and cookthe turkey frame until the remaining meat falls off the bones, about 1hour.
2. Remove the turkey carcass and remove and chop any remaining turkey meat. Chop the meat.
3. Strain the broth through a fine mesh strainer into a clean soup pot.Add the chopped turkey to the strained broth; bring the to a boil, reduce heat, and stir in the potatoes, carrots, celery, onion, cabbage,tomatoes, barley, Worcestershire sauce, salt, parsley, basil, bay leaf,black pepper, paprika, poultry seasoning, and thyme.
4. Simmer until the vegetables are tender, about 1 more hour.
5. Remove bay leaf before serving.

NUTRITION FACTS
Calories: 133 | Carbohydrates: 27.7g | Fat: 1.3g |
Protein: 4.2g |Cholesterol: 2mg

Pesto Green Vegetable Soup

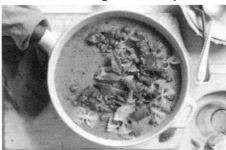

Preparation Time: 10 minutes
Cooking Time: 15 minutes
Servings: 6
Ingredients:

- 2 teaspoons olive oil
- 1 leek, sliced and washed thoroughly
- 2 celery stalks, diced
- 1 teaspoon minced garlic
- 2 cups sodium-free chicken stock
- 1 cup chopped snow peas
- 1 cup shredded spinach
- 1 tablespoon chopped fresh thyme
- Juice and zest of ½ lemon
- ¼ teaspoon freshly ground black pepper
- 1 tablespoon Basil Pesto

Directions:
1. Warm-up olive oil in a saucepan over medium-high heat. Add the leek, celery, and garlic, and sauté until tender, about 3 minutes.
2. Mix in the stock, and boil. Stir in the snow peas, spinach, and thyme, and simmer for about 5 minutes.
3. Remove the pan from the heat, and stir in the lemon juice, lemon zest, pepper, and pesto. Serve immediately.

Nutrition:

Calories: 170
Fat: 13 g
Sodium: 333 mg
Carbs: 8 g
Protein: 3 g
Phosphorus 181 mg
Potassium 1 mg

Vegetable Minestrone

Preparation Time: 20 minutes
Cooking Time: 20 minutes
Servings: 6
Ingredients:

- 1 teaspoon olive oil
- ½ sweet onion, chopped
- 1 celery stalk, diced
- 1 teaspoon minced garlic
- 2 cups sodium-free chicken stock
- 2 medium tomatoes, chopped
- 1 zucchini, diced
- ½ cup shredded stemmed kale
- Freshly ground black pepper
- 1-ounce grated Parmesan cheese

Directions:
1. Warm-up olive oil in a large saucepan over medium-high heat. Add the onion, celery, and garlic, and sauté until softened, about 5 minutes.
2. Stir in the stock, tomatoes, and zucchini, and boil. Adjust the heat to low, and simmer within 15 minutes. Stir in the kale and season with pepper. Garnish with the Parmesan cheese, and serve.

Nutrition:
Calories: 100
Fat: 3 g
Sodium: 195 mg
Carbs: 6 g
Protein: 4 g
Phosphorus 51 mg
Potassium 216 mg

Spinach Soup

Preparation Time: 15 minutes
Cooking Time: 30 minutes
Servings: 4
Ingredients:
- 1 tablespoon olive oil
- ½ sweet onion, chopped
- 2 teaspoons minced garlic
- 4 cups fresh spinach
- ¼ cup chopped fresh parsley
- 3 cups of water
- ¼ cup heavy (whipping) cream
- 1 tablespoon freshly squeezed lemon juice
- Freshly ground black pepper

Directions:
1. Warm-up olive oil in a large saucepan over medium-high heat. Put the onion plus garlic, and sauté within 3 minutes.
2. Add the spinach and parsley, and sauté for 5 minutes. Stir in the water, bring to a boil, and then reduce the heat to low. Simmer the soup within 20 minutes.
3. Cool the soup for about 5 minutes. Then, along with the heavy cream, purée the soup in batches your food processor or a blender, or with a handheld immersion blender.
4. Put the soup in the pot, and warm through on low heat. Add the lemon juice, season with pepper, and stir to combine. Serve hot.

Nutrition:
Calories: 141
Fat: 14 g
Sodium: 36 mg
Carbs: 3 g
Protein: 2 g
Phosphorus 50 mg
Potassium 300.8 mg

Carrot Soup

Preparation Time: 15 minutes
Cooking Time: 25 minutes
Servings: 4

Ingredients:

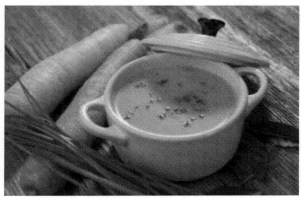

- 1 tablespoon olive oil
- ½ sweet onion, chopped
- 2 teaspoons grated peeled fresh ginger
- 1 teaspoon minced fresh garlic
- 4 cups of water
- 3 carrots, chopped
- 1 teaspoon ground turmeric
- ½ cup of coconut milk
- 1 tablespoon chopped fresh cilantro

Directions:
1. Warm-up olive oil in a large saucepan over medium-high heat. Sauté the onion, ginger, plus garlic within 3 minutes.
2. Mix in the water, carrots, plus turmeric. Boil the soup, adjust the heat to low, and simmer within 20 minutes.
3. Transfer the soup into a food processor or blender, and process with the coconut milk until the soup is smooth. Put the soup in the pan and reheat. Serve topped with the cilantro.

Nutrition:
Calories: 113
Fat: 10 g
Sodium: 30 mg
Carbs: 7 g
Protein: 7 g
Potassium 771 mg
Phosphorus 0 mg

Beef Stroganoff Soup

Preparation Time: 20 minutes
Cooking Time: 40 minutes
Servings: 6
Ingredients:

- 2 large beef rump (sirloin) steaks
- 600 g brown or white mushrooms, sliced
- ¼ cup of ghee or lard
- 2 cloves garlic, minced
- 1 medium white or brown onion, chopped
- 5 cups bone broth
- 2 teaspoons of paprika
- 1 tablespoon of Dijon mustard
- Juice from 1 lemon
- 1½ cup sour cream
- ¼ cup of freshly chopped parsley
- 1 teaspoon of salt
- ¼ teaspoon of freshly ground black pepper

Directions:

1. Lay the steaks in the freezer in a single layer for 30 to 45 minutes. Slice the steaks thinly using a sharp knife, then flavor it with some salt plus pepper.
2. Oiled a large, heavy bottom pan with half of the ghee and heat. Then, add the beef slices in a single layer. Do not overcrowd the pan.
3. Fry over medium-high heat until it's cooked through. Remove the slices, then place them in a bowl to set aside for later. Do the same for the remaining pieces.
4. Grease the pan with the remaining ghee. Put in the chopped onion plus minced garlic in the pan and cook until lightly browned and fragrant.
5. Put the sliced mushrooms and cook within 3 to 4 more minutes while stirring occasionally. Then add your Dijon mustard, paprika, and pour in the bone broth.
6. Add lemon juice and boil for 2 to 3 minutes, then put the browned beef slices plus sour cream. Remove from heat. If you are using a thickener, add it to the pot and stir well. Finally, add freshly chopped parsley. Enjoy!

Nutrition:
Calories: 0
Fat: 0 g
Sodium: 783 mg
Carbs: 10.8 g
Protein: 0 g
Phosphorus 289 mg
Potassium 663.4 mg

Chicken Stew

Preparation time: 5 minutes
Cooking time: 2 hours
Servings: 4
Ingredients:

- 2 cups of chicken stock
- 2 medium carrots, peeled and finely diced
- 2 celery sticks, diced
- ½ onion, diced
- 28 ounces skinless and deboned chicken thighs chopped into 1" pieces
- 1 fresh spring rosemary or ½ teaspoon dried rosemary
- 3 garlic cloves, minced
- ¼ teaspoon of dried thyme
- ½ teaspoon of dried oregano
- 1 cup of fresh spinach
- ½ cup of heavy cream
- salt and pepper, to taste
- xantham gum, to desired thickness starting at 1/8 teaspoon

Directions:

1. In a 3-quart crockpot, place the chicken stock, carrots, celery, onion, chicken thighs, rosemary, garlic, thyme, and oregano.
2. Cook on low within 4 hours or on high for 2 hours. Add salt and pepper to taste. Stir in spinach and the heavy cream.
3. Sprinkle and thicken with xantham gum to desired thickness starting at 1/8 teaspoon. Continue to whisk until mix and cook for another 10 minutes. Serve and enjoy.

Nutrition:

Calories: 228
Fat: 11 g
Sodium: 0 mg
Carbs: 6 g
Protein: 23 g
Phosphorus 114.4 mg
Potassium 0.25 mg

Chicken Fajita Soup

Preparation Time: 10 minutes
Cooking Time: 6 hours and 30 minutes
Servings: 8
Ingredients:

- 2 pounds of boneless skinless chicken breasts
- 1 cup of chicken broth
- 1 onion chopped
- 1 green pepper chopped
- 3 garlic cloves minced
- 1 tablespoon of Fat free butter or coconut spread
- 6 ounces of cream cheese
- 2 10 ounces of cans diced tomatoes with green chilis
- 2½ cups of chicken broth
- ½ cup of heavy whipping cream
- 2½ tablespoons of taco seasoning
- salt and pepper to taste

Directions:
1. Add boneless skinless chicken breasts to a slow cooker and cook within 3 hours on high or 6 hours on low. Flavor it with salt and pepper.
2. Remove the chicken and shred. In a large saucepan, fry green pepper, onion, and garlic in 1 tablespoon of Fat free butter or coconut spread until they are translucent (2 to 3 minutes).
3. Mash the cream cheese into the veggies with a spoon to combine smoothly as it melts. Add the canned tomatoes, chicken broth, heavy whipping cream, and taco seasoning.

4. Cook on low uncovered for 20 minutes. Put the chicken, cover, and cook within 10 minutes, then flavor it with salt and pepper to taste. Serve and enjoy!

Nutrition:
Calories: 306
Fat: 17 g
Sodium: 880 mg
Carbs: 8.2 g
Protein: 26 g
Phosphorus 106 mg
Potassium 303.2 mg

Italian Wedding Soup

Preparation time: 15 minutes
Cooking time: 25 minutes
Servings: 6
Ingredients:
Meatballs:

- 1 pound of ground beef or ground pork
- ½ cup of crushed pork rinds or almond flour
- ½ cup of grated parmesan cheese
- 1 teaspoon of Italian seasoning
- ¾ teaspoon of salt
- ½ teaspoon of pepper
- 1 large egg

Soup:

- 2 tablespoons of avocado oil
- ¼ cup of chopped onion
- 4 celery stalks chopped
- 1 teaspoon of salt
- ½ teaspoon of pepper
- 3 cloves garlic minced
- 1 teaspoon of dried oregano
- 6 cups of chicken broth
- 2 cups of riced cauliflower
- 2 cups of packed spinach leaves
- Additional salt and pepper
- Parmesan for sprinkling

Directions:

1. Mix the ground meat, crushed pork rinds, cheese, Italian seasoning, salt, plus pepper in a large mixing bowl. Put the egg and mix using your hands.
2. Form into ½ inch meatballs and place on a waxed paper-lined tray. Refrigerate until soup is ready. Warm-up oil over medium heat until shimmering in a large saucepan or stockpot.
3. Put the onion, celery, salt, pepper, and fry until vegetables are soft and tender within 7 minutes. Put the garlic and cook within 1 minute.
4. Stir in the chicken broth and oregano and simmer for 10 minutes, then put the cauliflower rice and meatballs and cook for about 5 minutes. Put the spinach leaves and cook within 2 minutes more. Season to taste. Serve and enjoy.

Nutrition:
Calories: 303
Fat: 20.16 g
Sodium: 0 mg
Carbs: 5.73 g
Protein: 29.48 g
Phosphorus 0 mg
Potassium 0 mg

Cream of Chicken Soup

Preparation time: 10 minutes
Cooking time: 20 minutes
Servings: 2
Ingredients:
- 2 cups of cauliflower florets
- 2/3 cup of unsweetened original almond milk
- 1 cup of chicken broth
- 1 teaspoon of onion powder
- ½ teaspoon of grey sea salt
- ¼ teaspoon of garlic powder
- ¼ teaspoon of freshly ground black pepper
- 1/8 teaspoon of celery seed (optional)
- 1/8 teaspoon of dried thyme
- ¼ cup of Beef Gelatin
- ¼ cup of finely diced cooked chicken thighs

Directions:
1. Place all ingredients but cook chicken and gelatin in a small saucepan. Boil over medium heat. Turn heat to low and cook within 7 to 8 minutes, until cauliflower is softened.
2. Remove from the heat. Add ½ cup or so of the hot liquid to a medium-sized bowl using a spoon. Add gelatin, one scoop at a time. Stir until dissolved, then add the next scoop.
3. Transfer the cauliflower mixture and gelatin mixture to your food processor, immersion blender, or high-powered blender. Blend until totally smooth.
4. Add cauliflower and gelatin mixture back to the saucepan. Add cooked chicken to cauliflower and gelatin mixture. Cover and heat on low within 2 to 5 minutes, until it thickens. Serve immediately. Enjoy friend.

Nutrition:
Calories: 198
Fat: 6.9 g
Sodium: 672 mg
Carbs: 9.4 g
Protein: 26.4 g
Phosphorus 0 mg
Potassium 0 mg

Green Chicken Enchilada Soup

Preparation time: 10 minutes
Cooking time: 5 minutes
Servings: 4
Ingredients:
- ½ cup of salsa Verde
- 4 ounces of cream cheese, softened
- 1 cup of sharp cheddar cheese, shredded
- 2 cups of bone broth
- 2 cups of cooked chicken, shredded

Directions:
1. Add the salsa, cream cheese, cheddar cheese, and chicken stock in a blender and blend until smooth. Put it into a medium saucepan and cook on medium until hot.

2. Add the shredded chicken and cook an additional 3 to 5 minutes until heated through. Garnish with extra shredded cheddar and chopped cilantro if desired. Enjoy.

Nutrition:
Calories: 346
Fat: 22 g
Sodium: 0 mg
Carbs: 3 g
Protein: 32 g
Potassium 547 mg
Phosphorus 0 mg

Bacon Cheeseburger Soup

Cooking time: 40 minutes
Preparation time: 20 minutes
Servings: 4
Ingredients:

- 5 slices bacon
- 12 ounces of ground beef (80/20)
- 2 tablespoons of Fat free butter or coconut spread
- 3 cups of beef broth
- ½ teaspoon of garlic powder
- ½ teaspoon of onion powder
- 2 teaspoons of brown mustard
- 1½ teaspoon of kosher salt
- ½ teaspoon of black pepper
- ½ teaspoon of red pepper flakes
- 1 teaspoon of cumin
- 1 teaspoon of chili powder
- 2½ tablespoons of tomato paste
- 1 medium dill pickle, diced
- 1 cup of shredded cheddar cheese
- 3 ounces of cream cheese
- ½ cup of heavy cream

Directions:
1. Start with cooking the bacon in a pan until crispy, then set aside. Add ground beef in the bacon fat and cook until browned on one side; flip and cook the other side until brown.
2. Place beef in a pot, and move it to the sides. Add Fat free butter or coconut spread and spices to the pan and let the spices sweat for 30 to 45 seconds.
3. Then add beef broth, tomato paste, mustard, cheese, and pickles to the pot and cook for a few minutes until it melts. Cover pot and turn to low heat.
4. Cook for another 20 to 30 minutes. Turn stove off, then finish with heavy cream and crumbled bacon. Stir well and serve. Enjoy.

Nutrition:
Calories: 48
Fat: 3.4 g
Sodium: 0 mg
Carbs: 0 g
Protein: 23.4 g
Phosphorus 181.8 mg
Potassium 0.28 mg

Roasted Garlic Soup

Preparation time: 10 minutes
Cooking time: 55 minutes
Servings: 6
Ingredients:

- 2 bulbs of garlic
- 1 tbsp extra-virgin olive oil, divided
- 3 shallots, chopped
- 1 large head of cauliflower, chopped
- 6 cups of gluten-free vegetable broth
- ¾ teaspoon of sea salt
- Freshly ground pepper, to taste

Directions:
1. First heat oven to 400F. Slice off the garlic bulb about ¼-inch from the top of the bulb. Put in on a square of aluminum foil, then coat each with ½ teaspoon of olive oil.
2. Heat in the oven within 35 minutes. Let it cool slightly before removing from aluminum foil. Squeeze out the garlic from each clove.

3. Drizzle the rest of your olive oil in a medium-sized saucepan. Turn heat to medium-high and add chopped shallots. Fry until tender for about 6 minutes.
4. In the saucepan, add the roasted garlic along with the remaining ingredients. Boil, then adjust the heat to low and cook for 15 to 20 minutes until the cauliflower is tender.
5. Drop mixture into the bowl of your blender. Puree until smooth, about 30 seconds. Adjust with salt and pepper and serve. Enjoy.

Nutrition:
Calories: 178.9
Fat: 9.1 g
Sodium: 1103.4 mg
Carbs: 19 g
Protein: 6.7 g
Phosphorus 13 mg
Potassium 32.8 mg

Cream of Crab Soup

Preparation Time: 10 minutes
Cooking Time: 30 minutes
Servings: 7
Ingredients:
- 1 tablespoon of unsalted Fat free butter or coconut spread
- 1 cup of onion
- ½ pound of fresh lump crab meat
- 4 cups of low-sodium chicken broth
- 1 cup of liquid non-dairy creamer
- 2 tablespoons of cornstarch
- 1/8 teaspoon of dill weed
- 1/8 teaspoon of Old Bay Seasoning
- 1/8 teaspoon of black pepper

Directions:
1. Dissolve the Fat free butter or coconut spread over medium heat in a large pot. Chop the onion and add it to the pot. Cook until the onion is soft.
2. Put the crab meat and cook for 2 to 3 minutes, stirring regularly. Add in the chicken

broth, bringing the mixture to a boil. Reduce the heat to low
3. Use a small bowl to combine the non-dairy creamer and cornstarch, then whisk until it becomes smooth. Add the mixture to the soup from step 4 and slightly increase the heat. Stir until it thickens. Add in the dill weed, Old Bay seasoning, and pepper to the soup. Serve.

Nutrition:
Calories 142
Protein 12g
Carbohydrates 10g
Fat 6g
Sodium 295mg
Potassium 244mg
Phosphorus 100mg

Rotisserie Chicken Noodle Soup

Preparation Time: 10 minutes
Cooking Time: 25 minutes
Servings: 10
Ingredients:
- 1 prepared rotisserie chicken
- 8 cups of low-sodium chicken broth
- ½ cup of onion
- 1 cup of celery
- 1 cup of carrots
- 6 ounces of uncooked wide noodles
- 3 tablespoons of fresh parsley

Directions:
1. Remove the chicken from the bones, chop into pieces of bite-sized, and measure 4 cups for the soup. Use a large stockpot and pour in the chicken broth, then bring to a boil
2. Chop the onion, and slice the celery and carrots. Put the chicken, vegetables, plus noodles to the stockpot, and bring to a boil. Cook within 15 minutes or until the noodles are done. Garnish with chopped parsley

Nutrition:
Calories 185

Protein 21g
Carbohydrates 14g
Fat 5g
Sodium 361mg
Potassium 294mg
Phosphorus 161mg

Irish Lamb Stew

Preparation Time: 10 minutes
Cooking Time: 1 hour & 35 minutes
Servings: 6
Ingredients:

- 1½ pounds of lamb shoulder, boneless
- ½ teaspoon of salt (or exclude to reduce sodium)
- ½ teaspoon of black pepper
- 1 tablespoon of olive oil
- 1 medium-sized onion
- ¼ cup of all-purpose flour
- 3 garlic cloves
- 1 teaspoon of dried thyme
- ½ cup of tomato sauce
- 1 cup of stout beer
- 2 cups of low-sodium beef broth
- 2 medium-sized carrots
- 2 medium-sized parsnips
- 1 cup of frozen green peas

Directions:

1. Cut lamb into 1 ½ chunk and dice the onion and garlic. Place the pieces of lamb on a plate, then sprinkle using salt and pepper. Place flour in a zip-top bag, add the lamb, then shake until meat is evenly coated.
2. Heat-up the one tablespoon of olive oil over medium heat in a Dutch oven or a large stockpot, add the lamb, then cook until it is browned evenly. Take it off from the pot and put aside
3. To the same pot, add the onion and fry until it is translucent. Add the diced garlic, stir for a minute, then add ½ cup of beef broth and stir to deglaze the pot.
4. Add the lamb, the remaining beef broth, tomato sauce, beer, and thyme to the pot. Reduce to low heat and cook. Simmer for 1 hour.
5. Cut into 1-inch pieces the carrots and parsnips, stir into the stew, then simmer for another 30 minutes. Add green peas, then cook for about 5 to 10 minutes.

Nutrition:
Calories 283
Protein 27g
Carbohydrates 19g
Fat 11g
Sodium 325mg
Potassium 527mg
Phosphorus 300mg

Creamy CarrotSoup

Preparation Time: 10 minutes
Cooking Time: 20 minutes
Servings: 5
Ingredients:

- 2 cups of low-sodium vegetable broth
- 3 cups of Carrotflorets
- 8 ounces of undrained silken tofu
- 3 tablespoons of cornstarch
- 3 tablespoons of nutritional yeast
- 1 teaspoon of onion powder
- 1 teaspoon of garlic powder
- ¼ teaspoon of black pepper
- 1/8 teaspoon of red pepper flakes

Directions:

1. Boil the Carrotflorets and tofu (including the liquid) in the vegetable broth using a large pot and cook until it is tender. Put aside to cool.
2. Pour the cooled contents into a large mixing bowl and use an immersion blender to blend until it becomes smooth.
3. Mix 1 ½ cups of the soup with the cornstarch in a small bowl, then whisk until it becomes smooth. Put the soup back into the pot, then put the mixed cornstarch and boil. Add the

nutritional yeast and all other spices, then stir until well combined.

Nutrition:
Calories 65
Protein 4g
Carbohydrates 10g
Fat 1g
Sodium 71mg
Potassium 289mg
Phosphorus 90mg

Southwestern Posole

Preparation Time: 10 minutes
Cooking Time: 50 minutes
Servings: 6
Ingredients:
- 1 tablespoon of olive oil
- 1 pound of pork loin
- ½ cup of onion
- 1 garlic clove
- 28 ounces canned of white hominy
- 4 ounces of canned diced green chilis
- 4 cups of low-sodium chicken broth
- ¼ teaspoon of black pepper

Directions:
1. Cut the pork into pieces of 1-inch, then chop the onion and the garlic. Drain and rinse the hominy. Using a skillet, heat oil over medium heat and brown the pieces of pork for about 3 to 4 minutes
2. Put the onion plus garlic in the skillet, then sauté until the onion is tender. Add the rest of the fixing and simmer for about 30 to 45 minutes. Serve.

Nutrition:
Calories 286
Protein 26g
Carbohydrates 15g
Fat 13g
Sodium 399mg
Potassium 346mg

Phosphorus 182mg

Red Lentil Dahl

Preparation Time: 10 minutes
Cooking Time: 30 minutes
Servings: 4
Ingredients:
- 1 cup of red lentils
- 1 tablespoon of canola oil
- ½ teaspoon of cumin seeds
- 1 2-inch of cinnamon stick
- 1 cup of diced yellow onion
- 1 green minced chili pepper
- 4 minced garlic cloves
- 1 tablespoon of minced ginger root
- ½ teaspoon of ground turmeric
- ½ teaspoon ground cardamom
- ½ teaspoon of paprika
- ¼ teaspoon of kosher salt (or exclude to reduce sodium)
- 1 medium-sized diced tomato
- 1½ juice of the lemon
- Chopped cilantro leaves

Directions:
To prepare the lentils:
1. Soak or dip the lentils in a bowl of water for about 12 hours or more. Rinse the lentils to get rid of the soaked water.
2. Using a medium-sized saucepan, add in the rinsed lentils along with 3 cups of water at room temperature, then boil over medium heat and cook for 20 minutes

To prepare the seasonings:
1. Using a medium-sized skillet, heat the canola oil over medium heat, add the cumin seeds, cinnamon stick, and cook for about 1 minute 30 seconds until it is fragrant.
2. Add in the onion, pepper, ginger, garlic, and cook for about 6 minutes until the onions become translucent.

3. Add in the turmeric, paprika, cardamom, salt, and tomato. Cook for about 3 minutes and discard the cinnamon stick
4. Once the lentils are ready, drain any extra water, and stir in the spiced onion mixture. Also, stir in the lemon juice. Garnish lentil soup with cilantro and serve with basmati rice

Nutrition:
Calories 230
Sodium 105 mg
Phosphorus 169mg
Potassium 32mg
Fats 0g
Protein 13g
Carbohydrates 37g

Shrimp and Crab Gumbo

Preparation Time: 10 minutes
Cooking Time: 25 minutes
Servings: 6
Ingredients:
- 1 cup of bell pepper
- 1½ cups of onion
- 1 garlic clove
- ¼ of cup celery leaves
- 1 cup of green onion tops
- ¼ cup of fresh parsley
- 4 tablespoons of canola oil
- 6 tablespoons of all-purpose white flour
- 3 cups of water
- 4 cups of low-sodium chicken broth
- 8 ounces of uncooked shrimp
- 6 ounces of crab meat
- ¼ teaspoon of black pepper
- 1 teaspoon of hot sauce
- 3 cups of cooked rice

Directions:
1. Chop the bell peppers, garlic, celery, onion, green onion tops, and parsley. For the roux, use a large skillet and heat oil and flour over medium heat. Stir until flour is color pecan.

2. Add in the bell peppers, onion, celery, garlic, and 1 cup of water. Cover and cook over low heat until the vegetables become tender.
3. Over high heat, add 2 cups of water and 4 cups of the low sodium chicken broth, then boil for about 5 minutes.
4. Over medium heat, add in the shrimp and crab meat, then boil for additional 10 minutes. Add in the green onion tops and parsley, then reduce the heat to low heat. Simmer for 5 minutes. Add pepper and hot sauce to the season, then serve with rice.

Nutrition:
Calories 327
Fat 11g
Protein 22g
Sodium 328mg
Fats 0g
Phosphorus 221mg
Potassium 368 mg
Carbohydrates 33g

Ground Beef Soup

Preparation Time: 15 minutes
Cooking Time: 35 minutes
Servings: 6
Ingredients:
- 1 pound of lean ground beef
- ½ cup of onion
- 2 teaspoons of Mrs. Dash lemon pepper
- 1 teaspoon of kitchen Bouquet seasoning and browning sauce
- 1 cup of reduced-sodium beef broth
- 2 cups of water
- 1/3 cup of uncooked brown rice
- 3 cups of frozen mixed vegetables (green beans, corn, peas, and carrots)
- 1 tablespoon of sour cream

Directions:
1. Slice the onion, brown the ground beef with the onion in a large saucepan, then drain fat. Add in the seasoning and browning sauce,

beef broth, water, rice, and the mixed vegetables.
2. Boil over high heat, reduce heat to medium-low, cover, and cook for about 30 minutes. Take off from heat, and stir in the sour cream. Serve.

Nutrition:
Calories 222
Protein 20g
Fat 8g
Sodium 170mg
Potassium 448mg
Phosphorus 210mg
Carbohydrates 204g

Yucatan Chicken Lime Soup

Preparation Time: 15 minutes
Cooking Time: 30 minutes
Servings: 4
Ingredients:
- ½ cup of onion
- 8 cloves of garlic
- 2 Serrano chili peppers
- 1 medium-sized tomato
- 1½ cups of uncooked chicken breast
- 2 (6-inch) corn tortillas
- Non-stick cooking spray
- 1 tablespoon of olive oil
- 4 cups of low-sodium chicken broth
- ¼ of teaspoon salt (or exclude to reduce sodium)
- 1 bay leaf
- ¼ cup of lime juice
- ¼ cup of fresh cilantro
- ½ teaspoon of black pepper

Directions:
1. Warm oven to 400° F. Slice the onion and cilantro, then mince the garlic cloves. Slice the chili peppers, and cut the tomato into half, and remove its skin and seeds. Shred the chicken.

2. Cut into strips the tortillas, and arrange it on a baking sheet. Oiled with cooking spray, then bake within 3 minutes or until it becomes slightly toasted. Take off from the oven, placing it on a plate to cool.
3. Heat-up the oil over medium heat in a large saucepan, h. Add the onion, garlic, and chili peppers, then cook until the onions become translucent.
4. Add the tomato, broth, chicken breast, bay leaf, and salt. Simmer for about 8 to 10 minutes. Add the lime juice and the fresh cilantro, then season using the black pepper. Taste, and add extra juice if desired. Serve and top with strips of tortilla.

Nutrition:
Calories 214
Protein 20g
Carbohydrates 12g
Fat 10g
Sodium 246mg
Potassium 355mg
Phosphorus 176mg

Beef and Barley Stew

Preparation Time: 20 minutes
Cooking Time: 1 hour & 35 minutes
Servings: 6
Ingredients:
- 1 cup of uncooked pearl barley
- 1 pound of lean beef stew meat
- 2 tablespoons of all-purpose white flour
- ¼ teaspoon of black pepper
- ¼ teaspoon of salt (or exclude to reduce sodium)
- 2 tablespoons of canola oil
- ½ cup of onion
- 1 large stalk celery
- 1 garlic clove
- 2 medium-sized carrots
- 2 bay leaves

- 1 teaspoon of Mrs. Dash onion herb seasoning

Directions:
1. Place the barley in 2 cups of water and soak for an hour. Dice the onion and celery, mince the garlic clove, slice the carrots into ¼-inch thick, and cut the beef into cubes of 1½inch.
2. Place flour in a zip-top bag, add black pepper, and stew meat, then shake until the meat is evenly coated. Heat oil using a 4-quart pot and brown the stew meat. Take the stew meat off the pot
3. Sauté and stir in meat drippings the onion, celery, and garlic for 2 minutes, then add 2 quarts of water and boil. Put the meat in the pot, add salt and bay leaves, and reduce the heat to a simmer.
4. Drain and rinse the barley, pour into the pot, cover, and then cook for 1 hour. Stirring every 15 minutes. After 1 hour, add carrots and Mrs. Dash seasoning. Simmer for about 30 minutes. Add extra water if necessary to prevent sticking

Nutrition:
Calories 246
Protein 22g
Carbohydrates 21g
Fat 8g
Sodium 222mg
Potassium 369mg
Phosphorus 175mg

Beef and Cabbage Borscht Soup

Preparation Time: 15 minutes
Cooking Time: 2 hours
Servings: 12
Ingredients:
- 2 pounds of beef blade steaks
- 6 cups of cold water
- 2 tablespoons of olive oil
- ½ cup of low-sodium tomato sauce
- 1 medium-sized cabbage
- 1 cup of onion
- 1 cup of carrots
- 1 cup of turnips
- ¾ teaspoon of salt (or exclude to reduce sodium)
- 1 teaspoon of pepper
- tablespoons of lemon juice
- 4 tablespoons of stevia or aspartame

Directions:
1. Place the steak in a large pot, add water to cover the meat, cover, and boil. When the water boil, reduce the heat to simmer, then cook until the meat becomes tender
2. Take the meat off the pot, shredding with a fork. Cut the cabbage into pieces of bite-size, diced onion, carrots, and turnips.
3. With the meat broth still in the pot, add the olive oil, tomato sauce, cabbage, carrots, turnips, onion, and shredded meat. Put salt plus pepper to season, then add the lemon juice and sugar.
4. Allow cooking on low heat for about 1 to 1½hours until all the vegetables are well cooked. Taste for seasoning, adding extra lemon, sugar, or pepper if desired

Nutrition:
Calories 202
Protein 19g
Carbohydrates 9g
Fat 10g
Sodium 242mg
Potassium 388mg
Phosphorus 160mg

Broths, Condiment and Seasoning Mix

Spicy Herb Seasoning

Preparation time: 10 minutes
Cooking time: 0 minutes
Servings: ½ cup
Ingredients:

- ¼ cup celery seed
- 1 tablespoon dried basil
- 1 tablespoon dried oregano
- 1 tablespoon dried thyme
- 1 tablespoon onion powder
- 2 teaspoons garlic powder
- 1 teaspoon freshly ground black pepper
- ½ teaspoon ground cloves

Directions:
1. Mix the celery seed, basil, oregano, thyme, onion powder, garlic powder, pepper, and cloves in a small bowl. Store for up to 1 month.

Nutrition:
Calories: 7
Fat: 0g
Sodium: 2mg
Carbohydrates: 1g
Phosphorus: 9mg
Potassium: 27mg
Protein: 0g

Phosphorus-Free Baking Powder

Preparation time: 5 minutes
Cooking time: 0 minutes
Servings: 1
Ingredients:

- ¾ cup cream of tartar
- ¼ cup baking soda

Directions:
1. Mix the cream of tartar plus baking soda in a small bowl. Sift the mixture together several times to mix thoroughly. Store the baking powder in a sealed container in a cool, dark place for up to 1 month.

Nutrition:
Calories: 6
Fat: 0g
Sodium: 309mg
Carbohydrates: 1g
Phosphorus: 0g
Potassium: 341mg
Protein: 0g

Basil Oil

Preparation time: 15 minutes
Cooking time: 4 minutes
Servings: 3
Ingredients:

- 2 cups olive oil
- 2½ cups fresh basil leaves patted dry

Directions:
1. Put the olive oil plus basil leaves in a food processor or blender, and pulse until the leaves are coarsely chopped.
2. Transfer these to a medium saucepan, and place over medium heat. Heat the oil, occasionally stirring, until it just starts to simmer along the edges, about 4 minutes. Remove, then let it stand until cool, about 2 hours.
3. Pour the oil through a fine-mesh sieve or doubled piece of cheesecloth into a container. Store the basil oil in an airtight glass container in the refrigerator for up to 2 months.
4. Before using for dressings, remove the oil from the refrigerator and let it come to room temperature or scoop out cold spoonsful for cooking.

Nutrition:
Calories: 40
Fat: 5g
Sodium: 0g
Carbohydrates: 0g

Phosphorus: 0g
Potassium: 0g
Protein: 0g

Tomatillo Salsa Verde

Servings: 8 | Prep: 10m | Cooks: 15m | Total: 25m

INGREDIENTS

1 pound tomatillos, husked
1 tablespoon chopped fresh oregano
1/2 cup finely chopped onion
1/2 teaspoon ground cumin
1 teaspoon minced garlic
1 1/2 teaspoons salt, or to taste
1 serrano chile peppers, minced
2 cups water
2 tablespoons chopped cilantro

DIRECTIONS

Place tomatillos, onion, garlic, and chile pepper into a saucepan.Season with cilantro, oregano, cumin, and salt; pour in water. Bringto a boil over high heat, then reduce heat to medium-low, and simmer until the tomatillos are soft, 10 to 15 minutes.

Using a blender, carefully puree the tomatillos and water inbatches until smooth

NUTRITION FACTS

Calories: 24 | Carbohydrates: 4.6g | Fat: 0.6g | Protein: 0.8g |Cholesterol: 0mg

Fresh Apple Sauce

Servings: 8 | Prep: 15m | Cooks: 30m | Total: 45m

INGREDIENTS

3 pounds apples - peeled, cored and chopped
1 cup white sugar
3 cups water
1 tablespoon lemon juice

DIRECTIONS

Place apples in a large saucepan and just barely cover with water.Simmer over medium-low heat until apples are tender, 15 to 20 minutes.

Run cooked apples through a food mill or blender. Stir in the sugarand lemon juice. Cook over medium heat for about 3 to 5 minutes.

NUTRITION FACTS

Calories: 186 | Carbohydrates: 48.6g | Fat: 0.3g | Protein: 0.5g |Cholesterol: 0mg

Basil Pesto

Preparation time: 15 minutes
Cooking time: 0 minutes
Servings: 1 ½ cups
Ingredients:

- 2 cups gently packed fresh basil leaves
- 2 garlic cloves
- 2 tablespoons pine nuts
- ¼ cup olive oil
- 2 tablespoons freshly squeezed lemon juice

Directions:
1. Pulse the basil, garlic, plus pine nuts using a food processor or blender within about 3 minutes. Drizzle the olive oil into this batter, and pulse until thick paste forms.
2. Put the lemon juice, and pulse until well blended. Store the pesto in a sealed glass container in the refrigerator for up to 2 weeks.

Nutrition:
Calories: 22
Fat: 2g
Sodium: 0mg
Carbohydrates: 0g
Phosphorus: 3mg
Potassium: 10mg
Protein: 0g

Sweet Barbecue Sauce

Preparation time: 15 minutes
Cooking time: 11 minutes
Servings: 2 cups
Ingredients:

- 1 teaspoon olive oil
- ½ sweet onion, chopped
- 1 teaspoon minced garlic
- ¼ cup honey
- ¼ cup apple cider vinegar
- 2 tablespoons low-sodium tomato paste
- 1 tablespoon Dijon mustard
- 1 teaspoon hot sauce
- 1 teaspoon cornstarch

Directions:
1. Warm-up olive oil in a medium saucepan over medium heat. Add the onion and garlic and sauté until softened, about 3 minutes.
2. Stir in ¾ cup water, the honey, vinegar, tomato paste, mustard, and hot sauce. Cook within 6 minutes.
3. In a small cup, stir together ¼ cup of water and the cornstarch. Whisk the cornstarch into the sauce and continue to cook, stirring until it thickens about 2 minutes. Cool. Pour the sauce into a sealed glass container and store in the refrigerator for up to 1 week.

Nutrition:
Calories: 14
Fat: 0g
Sodium: 10mg
Carbohydrates: 3g
Phosphorus: 3mg
Potassium: 17mg
Protein: 0g

Low-Sodium Mayonnaise

Preparation time: 15 minutes
Cooking time: 0 minutes
Servings: 3
Ingredients:

- 2 egg yolks
- 1 teaspoon Dijon mustard
- 1 teaspoon honey
- 2 tablespoons white vinegar
- 2 tablespoons freshly squeezed lemon juice
- 2 cups olive oil

Directions:
1. Mix the egg yolks, mustard, honey, vinegar, and lemon juice in a large bowl. Mix in the olive oil in a thin stream. You can store this in a glass container in the refrigerator for up to 2 weeks.

Nutrition:
Calories: 83
Fat: 9g
Sodium: 2mg
Carbohydrates: 0g
Phosphorus: 2mg
Potassium: 3mg
Protein: 0g

Citrus and Mustard Marinade

Preparation time: 15 minutes
Cooking time: 0 minutes
Servings: ¾ cup
Ingredients:

- ¼ cup freshly squeezed lemon juice
- ¼ cup freshly squeezed orange juice
- ¼ cup Dijon mustard
- 2 tablespoons honey
- 2 teaspoons chopped fresh thyme

Directions:
1. Mix the lemon juice, orange juice, mustard, honey, and thyme until well blended in a medium bowl. Store the marinade in a sealed glass container in the refrigerator for up to 3 days. Shake before using it.

Nutrition:
Calories: 35
Fat: 0g

Sodium: 118mg
Carbohydrates: 8g
Phosphorus: 14mg
Potassium: 52mg
Protein: 1g

Fiery Honey Vinaigrette

Preparation time: 15 minutes
Cooking time: 0 minutes
Servings: ¾ cup
Ingredients:

- 1/3 cup freshly squeezed lime juice
- ¼ cup honey
- ¼ cup olive oil
- 1 teaspoon chopped fresh basil leaves
- ½ teaspoon red pepper flakes

Directions:
1. Mix the lime juice, honey, olive oil, basil, and red pepper flakes in a medium bowl, until well blended. Store the dressing in a glass container, and store it in the fridge for up to 1 week.

Nutrition:
Calories: 125
Fat: 1.1g
Sodium: 1mg
Carbohydrates: 13g
Phosphorus: 1mg
Potassium: 24mg
Protein: 0g

Fat Free Milky Herb Dressing

Preparation time: 15 minutes
Cooking time: 0 minutes
Servings: 1 ½ cup
Ingredients:

- ½ cup low fat milk
- ½ cup Low-Sodium Mayonnaise
- 2 tablespoons apple cider vinegar
- ½ scallion, green part only, chopped
- 1 tablespoon chopped fresh dill

- 1 teaspoon chopped fresh thyme
- ½ teaspoon minced garlic
- Freshly ground black pepper

Directions:
1. Mix the milk, mayonnaise, and vinegar until smooth in a medium bowl. Whisk in the scallion, dill, thyme, and garlic. Season with pepper. Store.

Nutrition:
Calories: 31
Fat: 1,5g
Sodium: 19mg
Carbohydrates: 2g
Phosphorus: 13mg
Potassium: 26mg
Protein: 0g

Poppy Seed Dressing

Preparation time: 15 minutes
Cooking time: 0 minutes
Servings: 2 cups
Ingredients:

- ½ cup apple cider or red wine vinegar
- 1/3 cup honey
- ¼ cup freshly squeezed lemon juice
- 1 tablespoon Dijon mustard
- 1 cup olive oil
- ½ small sweet onion, minced
- 2 tablespoons poppy seeds

Directions:
1. Mix the vinegar, honey, lemon juice, and mustard in a small bowl. Whisk in the oil, onion, and poppy seeds. Store the dressing in a sealed glass container in the refrigerator for up to 2 weeks.

Nutrition:
Calories: 151
Fat: 14g
Sodium: 12mg
Carbohydrates: 7g

Phosphorus: 13mg
Potassium: 30mg
Protein: 0g

Mediterranean Dressing

Preparation time: 15 minutes
Cooking time: 0 minutes
Servings: 1 cup
Ingredients:

- ½ cup balsamic vinegar
- 1 teaspoon honey
- ½ teaspoon minced garlic
- 1 tablespoon dried parsley
- 1 tablespoon dried oregano
- ½ teaspoon celery seed
- Pinch freshly ground black pepper
- ½ cup olive oil

Directions:
1. Mix the vinegar, honey, garlic, parsley, oregano, celery seed, and pepper in a small bowl. Whisk in the olive oil until emulsified. Store the dressing in a sealed glass container in the refrigerator for up to 1 week.

Nutrition:
Calories: 100
Fat: 11g
Sodium: 1mg
Carbohydrates: 1g
Phosphorus: 1mg
Potassium: 10mg
Protein: 0g

Slow Cooker Mediterranean Stew

Servings: 10 | Prep: 30m | Cooks: 10h | Total: 10h30m

INGREDIENTS
1 butternut squash - peeled, seeded, and cubed
1/2 cup vegetable broth
2 cups cubed eggplant, with peel
1/3 cup raisins
2 cups cubed zucchini

1 clove garlic, chopped
1 (10 ounce) package frozen okra, thawed
1/2 teaspoon ground cumin
1 (8 ounce) can tomato sauce
1/2 teaspoon ground turmeric
1 cup chopped onion
1/4 teaspoon crushed red pepper
1 ripe tomato, chopped
1/4 teaspoon ground cinnamon
1 carrot, sliced thin
1/4 teaspoon paprika

DIRECTIONS
In a slow cooker, combine butternut squash, eggplant, zucchini, okra, tomato sauce, onion, tomato, carrot, broth, raisins, and garlic.Season with cumin, turmeric, red pepper, cinnamon, and paprika.
Cover, and cook on Low for 8 to 10 hours, or until vegetables aretender.

NUTRITION FACTS
Calories: 122 | Carbohydrates: 30.5g | Fat: 0.5g | Protein: 3.4g | Cholesterol: 0mg

Fajita Rub

Preparation time: 15 minutes
Cooking time: 0 minutes
Servings: ¼ cup
Ingredients:

- 1½ teaspoons chili powder
- 1 teaspoon garlic powder
- 1 teaspoon roasted cumin seed
- 1 teaspoon dried oregano
- ½ teaspoon ground coriander
- ¼ teaspoon red pepper flakes

Directions:
1. Put the chili powder, garlic powder, cumin seed, oregano, coriander, and red pepper flakes in a blender, pulse until ground and well combined. Transfer the spice mixture and store for up to 6 months.

Nutrition:

Calories: 1
Fat: 0g
Carbohydrates: 0g
Phosphorus: 2mg
Potassium: 7mg
Sodium: 7mg
Protein: 0g

Dried Herb Rub

Preparation time: 15 minutes
Cooking time: 0 minutes
Servings: 1/3 cup
Ingredients:

- 1 tablespoon dried thyme
- 1 tablespoon dried oregano
- 1 tablespoon dried parsley
- 2 teaspoons dried basil
- 2 teaspoons ground coriander
- 2 teaspoons onion powder
- 1 teaspoon ground cumin
- 1 teaspoon garlic powder
- 1 teaspoon paprika
- ½ teaspoon cayenne pepper

Directions:
1. Put the thyme, oregano, parsley, basil, coriander, onion powder, cumin, garlic powder, paprika, and cayenne pepper in a blender, and pulse until the ingredients are ground and well combined. Transfer the rub to a small container with a lid. Store in a cool, dry area for up to 6 months.

Nutrition:
Calories: 3
Fat: 0g
Carbohydrates: 1g
Phosphorus: 3mg
Potassium: 16mg
Sodium: 1mg
Protein: 0g

Mediterranean Seasoning

Preparation time: 15 minutes
Cooking time: 0 minutes
Servings: 1
Ingredients:

- 2 tablespoons dried oregano
- 1 tablespoon dried thyme
- 2 teaspoons dried rosemary, chopped finely or crushed
- 2 teaspoons dried basil
- 1 teaspoon dried marjoram
- 1 teaspoon dried parsley flakes

Directions:
1. Mix the oregano, thyme, rosemary, basil, marjoram, and parsley in a small bowl until well combined. Transfer then store.

Nutrition:
Calories: 1
Fat: 0g
Carbohydrates: 0g
Phosphorus: 1mg
Potassium: 6mg
Sodium: 0mg
Protein: 0g

Hot Curry Powder

Preparation time: 15 minutes
Cooking time: 0 minutes
Servings: 1 ¼ cup
Ingredients:

- ¼ cup ground cumin
- ¼ cup ground coriander
- 3 tablespoons turmeric
- 2 tablespoons sweet paprika
- 2 tablespoons ground mustard
- 1 tablespoon fennel powder
- ½ teaspoon green chili powder
- 2 teaspoons ground cardamom
- 1 teaspoon ground cinnamon
- ½ teaspoon ground cloves

Directions:
1. Pulse the cumin, coriander, turmeric, paprika, mustard, fennel powder, green chili powder, cardamom, cinnamon, plus cloves using a blender, until the fixing is ground and well combined. Transfer it to a small container, put in a cool, dry place for up to 6 months.

Nutrition:
Calories: 19
Fat: 1g
Carbohydrates: 3g
Phosphorus: 24mg
Potassium: 93mg
Sodium: 5mg
Protein: 1g

Cajun Seasoning
Preparation time: 15 minutes
Cooking time: 0 minutes
Servings: 1 ¼ cup
Ingredients:
- ½ cup sweet paprika
- ¼ cup garlic powder
- 3 tablespoons onion powder
- 3 tablespoons freshly ground black pepper
- 2 tablespoons dried oregano
- 1 tablespoon cayenne pepper
- 1 tablespoon dried thyme

Directions:
1. Pulse the paprika, garlic powder, onion powder, black pepper, oregano, cayenne pepper, and thyme in a blender until the fixing is ground and well combined.

Nutrition:
Calories: 7
Fat: 0g
Carbohydrates: 2g
Phosphorus: 8mg
Potassium: 40mg
Sodium: 1mg
Protein: 0g

Apple Pie Spice
Preparation time: 15 minutes
Cooking time: 0 minutes
Servings: 1/3 cup
Ingredients:
- ¼ cup ground cinnamon
- 2 teaspoons ground nutmeg
- 2 teaspoons ground ginger
- 1 teaspoon allspice
- ½ teaspoon ground cloves

Directions:
1. Mix the cinnamon, nutmeg, ginger, allspice, and cloves in a small bowl. Store for up to 6 months.

Nutrition:
Calories: 6
Fat: 0g
Carbohydrates: 1g
Phosphorus: 2mg
Potassium: 12mg
Sodium: 1mg
Protein: 0g

Ras El Hanout
Preparation time: 5 minutes
Cooking time: 0 minutes
Servings: ½ cup
Ingredients:
- 2 teaspoons ground nutmeg
- 2 teaspoons ground coriander
- 2 teaspoons ground cumin
- 2 teaspoons turmeric
- 2 teaspoons cinnamon
- 1 teaspoon cardamom
- 1 teaspoon sweet paprika
- 1 teaspoon ground mace
- 1 teaspoon freshly ground black pepper
- 1 teaspoon cayenne pepper
- ½ teaspoon ground allspice
- ½ teaspoon ground cloves

Directions:

1. Mix the nutmeg, coriander, cumin, turmeric, cinnamon, cardamom, paprika, mace, black pepper, cayenne pepper, allspice, and cloves in a small bowl. Store.

Nutrition:
Calories: 5
Fat: 0g
Carbohydrates: 1g
Phosphorus: 3mg
Potassium: 17mg
Sodium: 1mg
Protein: 0g

Poultry Seasoning

Preparation time: 15 minutes
Cooking time: 0 minutes
Servings: ½ cup
Ingredients:

- 2 tablespoons ground thyme
- 2 tablespoons ground marjoram
- 1 tablespoon ground sage
- 1 tablespoon ground celery seed
- 1 teaspoon ground rosemary
- 1 teaspoon freshly ground black pepper

Directions:

1. Mix the thyme, marjoram, sage, celery seed, rosemary, and pepper in a small bowl. Store for up to 6 months.

Nutrition:
Calories: 3
Fat: 0g
Carbohydrates: 0g
Phosphorus: 3mg
Potassium: 10mg
Sodium: 1mg
Protein: 0g

Berbere Spice Mix

Preparation time: 15 minutes
Cooking time: 4 minutes
Servings: ½ cup
Ingredients:

- 1 tablespoon coriander seeds
- 1 teaspoon cumin seeds
- 1 teaspoon fenugreek seeds
- ¼ teaspoon black peppercorns
- ¼ teaspoon whole allspice berries
- 4 whole cloves
- 4 dried chilis, stemmed and seeded
- ¼ cup dried onion flakes
- 2 tablespoons ground cardamom
- 1 tablespoon sweet paprika
- 1 teaspoon ground ginger
- ½ teaspoon ground nutmeg
- ½ teaspoon ground cinnamon

Directions:

1. Put the coriander, cumin, fenugreek, peppercorns, allspice, and cloves in a small skillet over medium heat. Lightly toast the spices, swirling the skillet frequently, for about 4 minutes or until the spices are fragrant.
2. Remove the skillet, then let the spices cool for about 10 minutes. Transfer the toasted spices to a blender with the chilis and onion, and grind until the mixture is finely ground.
3. Transfer the ground spice mixture to a small bowl and stir together the cardamom, paprika, ginger, nutmeg, and cinnamon until thoroughly combined. Store the spice mixture in a small container with a lid for up to 6 months.

Nutrition:
Calories: 8
Fat: 0g
Carbohydrates: 2g
Phosphorus: 7mg
Potassium: 37mg
Sodium: 14mg
Protein: 0g

Creole Seasoning Mix

Preparation time: 15 minutes
Cooking time: 0 minutes
Servings: ¼ cup

Ingredients:

- 1 tablespoon sweet paprika
- 1 tablespoon garlic powder
- 2 teaspoons onion powder
- 2 teaspoons dried oregano
- 1 teaspoon cayenne pepper
- 1 teaspoon ground thyme
- 1 teaspoon freshly ground black pepper

Directions:

1. Mix the paprika, garlic powder, onion powder, oregano, cayenne pepper, thyme, and black pepper in a small bowl. Store for up to 6 months.

Nutrition:
Calories: 7
Fat: 0g
Carbohydrates: 2g
Phosphorus: 8mg
Potassium: 35mg
Sodium: 1mg
Protein: 0g

Adobo Seasoning Mix

Preparation time: 15 minutes
Cooking time: 0 minutes
Servings: 1 ¼ cup
Ingredients:

- 4 tablespoons garlic powder
- 4 tablespoons onion powder
- 4 tablespoons ground cumin
- 3 tablespoons dried oregano
- 3 tablespoons freshly ground black pepper
- 2 tablespoons sweet paprika
- 2 tablespoons ground chili powder
- 1 tablespoon ground turmeric
- 1 tablespoon ground coriander

Directions:

1. Mix the garlic powder, onion powder, black pepper, cumin, oregano, paprika, chili powder, turmeric, and coriander in a small bowl. Transfer these to a container and store in a cool, dry place for up to 6 months.

Nutrition:
Calories: 8
Fat: 0g
Carbohydrates: 2g
Phosphorus: 9mg
Potassium: 38mg
Sodium: 12mg
Protein: 0g

Herbes De Provence

Preparation time: 15 minutes
Cooking time: 0 minutes
Servings: 1 cup
Ingredients:

- ½ cup dried thyme
- 3 tablespoons dried marjoram
- 3 tablespoons dried savory
- 2 tablespoons dried rosemary
- 2 teaspoons dried lavender flowers
- 1 teaspoon ground fennel

Directions:

1. Put the thyme, marjoram, savory, rosemary, lavender, and fennel in a blender and pulse a few times to combine. Store for up to 6 months.

Nutrition:
Calories: 3
Fat: 0g
Carbohydrates: 1g
Phosphorus: 2mg
Potassium: 9mg
Sodium: 0mg
Protein: 0g

Lamb and Pork Seasoning

Preparation time: 15 minutes
Cooking time: 0 minutes
Servings: ½ cup
Ingredients:

- ¼ cup celery seed
- 2 tablespoons dried oregano

- 2 tablespoons onion powder
- 1 tablespoon dried thyme
- 1½ teaspoons garlic powder
- 1 teaspoon crushed bay leaf
- 1 teaspoon freshly ground black pepper
- 1 teaspoon ground allspice

Directions:
1. Pulse the celery seed, oregano, onion powder, thyme, garlic powder, bay leaf, pepper, and allspice in a blender a few times. Transfer the herb mixture to a small container; then, you can store it in a cool, dry place for up to 6 months.

Nutrition:
Calories: 8
Fat: 0g
Carbohydrates: 1g
Phosphorus: 9mg
Potassium: 29mg
Sodium: 2mg

Asian Seasoning

Preparation time: 5 minutes
Cooking time: 0 minutes
Servings: ½ cup
Ingredients:
- 2 tablespoons sesame seeds
- 2 tablespoons onion powder
- 2 tablespoons crushed star anise pods
- 2 tablespoons ground ginger
- 1 teaspoon ground allspice
- ½ teaspoon cardamom
- ½ teaspoon ground cloves

Directions:
1. Mix the sesame seeds, onion powder, star anise, ginger, allspice, cardamom, and cloves in a small bowl. Transfer the spice mixture to a container with a cover. Store for up to 6 months.

Nutrition:

Calories: 10
Fat: 0g
Carbohydrates: 1g
Phosphorus: 11mg
Potassium: 24mg
Sodium: 5mg
Protein: 0g

Onion Seasoning Blend

Preparation time: 15 minutes
Cooking time: 0 minutes
Servings: ½ cup
Ingredients:
- 2 tablespoons onion powder
- 1 tablespoon dry mustard
- 2 teaspoons sweet paprika
- 2 teaspoons garlic powder
- 1 teaspoon dried thyme
- ½ teaspoon celery seeds
- ½ teaspoon freshly ground black pepper

Directions:
1. Mix the onion powder, mustard, paprika, garlic powder, thyme, celery seeds, and pepper until well combined in a small bowl. Store for up to 6 months.

Nutrition:
Calories: 5
Fat: 0g
Carbohydrates: 1g
Phosphorus: 6mg
Potassium: 17mg
Sodium: 1mg
Protein: 1g

Everyday No-Salt Seasoning Blend

Preparation time: 15 minutes
Cooking time: 0 minutes
Servings: 2 tbsp
Ingredients:
- 1 teaspoon dried thyme leaves
- 1 teaspoon dried marjoram leaves

- 1 teaspoon dried basil leaves
- 1 teaspoon dried oregano leaves
- ½ teaspoon onion powder
- ½ teaspoon garlic powder
- ½ teaspoon ground mustard
- ¼ teaspoon freshly ground black pepper
- ¼ teaspoon paprika

Directions:
1. Combine the thyme, marjoram, basil, oregano, onion powder, garlic powder, ground mustard, pepper, and paprika. Transfer and store at room temperature for up to 6 months.

Nutrition:
Calories: 4
Fat: 0g
Sodium: 0mg
Potassium: 17mg
Phosphorus: 4mg
Carbohydrates: 1g
Protein: 0g

Thai-Style Seasoning Blend

Preparation time: 15 minutes
Cooking time: 0 minutes
Servings: 3 tbsp
Ingredients:
- 1½ teaspoons turmeric
- 1½ teaspoons paprika
- 1 teaspoon ground coriander
- 1 teaspoon ground ginger
- 1 teaspoon dry mustard
- 1 teaspoon ground cumin
- 1 teaspoon dried mint leaves, crushed
- 1 teaspoon red pepper flakes

Directions:
1. Combine the turmeric, paprika, coriander, ginger, dry mustard, cumin, mint, and red pepper flakes and store for up to 6 months.

Nutrition:

Calories: 5
Fat: 0g
Sodium: 1mg
Potassium: 30mg
Phosphorus: 6mg
Carbohydrates: 1g
Protein: 0g

Tex-Mex Seasoning Mix

Preparation time: 10 minutes
Cooking time: 0 minutes
Servings: 2 tbsp
Ingredients:
- 1 tablespoon chili powder
- ½ teaspoon ground cumin
- ½ teaspoon dried oregano leaves
- ½ teaspoon garlic powder
- ½ teaspoon onion powder
- ½ teaspoon cayenne pepper
- ½ teaspoon red pepper flakes

Directions:
1. Combine the chili powder, cumin, oregano, garlic powder, onion powder, cayenne pepper, and red pepper flakes. Store for up to 6 months.

Nutrition:
Calories: 7
Fat: 0g
Sodium: 39mg
Potassium: 38mg
Phosphorus: 7mg
Carbohydrates: 1g
Protein: 0g

Duxelles

Preparation time: 15 minutes
Cooking time: 15 minutes
Servings: 8
Ingredients:
- 1 (8-ounce) package sliced cremini mushrooms

- 3 scallions, white and green parts
- 3 garlic cloves
- 1 tablespoon olive oil
- 1 tablespoon unsalted Fat free butter or coconut spread
- 1 teaspoon freshly squeezed lemon juice
- Pinch salt

Directions:
1. Finely chop the mushrooms, scallions, and garlic in a food processor or blender. Put the mushroom batter in the middle of a kitchen towel. Gather up the ends to create a pouch, and squeeze the pouch over the sink to remove some of the mushrooms' liquid.
2. Heat-up olive oil and Fat free butter or coconut spread in a large skillet over medium-high heat. Add the drained mushroom mixture to the skillet and sprinkle with the lemon juice and salt.
3. Sauté for 8 to 12 minutes, stirring frequently, or until the mushrooms are browned. This mixture can be refrigerated up to 4 days or frozen up to 1 month.

Nutrition:
Calories: 37
Fat: 3g
Sodium: 22mg
Potassium: 141mg
Phosphorus: 37mg
Carbohydrates: 2g
Protein: 1g

Chicken Stock

Preparation time: 15 minutes
Cooking time: 25 minutes
Servings: 4
Ingredients:
- 1 tablespoon olive oil
- 1 bone-in skin-on chicken breast (3 to 4 ounces)
- Pinch salt
- 1 onion, unpeeled, sliced

- 1 carrot, unpeeled, sliced
- 1 bay leaf
- 5 cups of water

Directions:
1. Heat-up olive oil in a large saucepan over medium-high heat. Sprinkle the chicken with salt and add to the pan, skin-side down. Brown for 2 minutes.
2. Put the onion plus carrot and cook within 1 minute longer. Add the bay leaf and water and bring to a boil. Adjust the heat to medium-low and simmer within 20 to 22 minutes, stirring occasionally. Remove the scum that pops to the surface.
3. Drain or strain the stock through a fine-mesh colander into a bowl. You can reserve the chicken breast for other recipes, although it may be tough after cooking. Discard the remaining solids.
4. Fridge the broth and skim off any fat that rises to the top. You can freeze this stock in 1-cup measures to use in recipes. Store freezer up to 3 months.

Nutrition:
Calories: 37
Fat: 2g
Sodium: 22mg
Potassium: 85mg
Phosphorus: 30mg
Carbohydrates: 2g
Protein: 3g

Vegetable Broth

Preparation time: 15 minutes
Cooking time: 27 minutes
Servings: 4
Ingredients:
- 1 tablespoon olive oil
- 1 unpeeled onion, sliced
- 2 unpeeled garlic cloves, crushed
- 2 unpeeled carrots, sliced
- 2 celery stalks, cut into 2-inch pieces

- 1 bay leaf
- 1 teaspoon dried basil leaves
- 5 cups of water

Directions:
1. Heat-up olive oil in a large saucepan over medium-high heat. Sauté the onion, garlic, carrot, and celery for 5 minutes, stirring frequently or lightly browned.
2. Add the bay leaf, basil, and water to the saucepan and bring to a boil. Adjust the heat to medium-low, then simmer for 20 to 22 minutes, stirring occasionally. Skim off and discard any scum that rises to the surface.
3. Strain the stock to a fine-mesh colander into a bowl. Discard the solids. Fridge the broth and remove any fat that rises to the top. You can freeze this broth in 1-cup measures to use in recipes.

Nutrition:
Calories: 31
Fat: 2g
Sodium: 21mg
Potassium: 110mg
Phosphorus: 14mg
Carbohydrates: 4g
Protein: 0g

Powerhouse Salsa

Preparation time: 15 minutes
Cooking time: 0 minutes
Servings: 8
Ingredients:
- 8 grape tomatoes, chopped
- 1 yellow bell pepper, chopped
- 1 red bell pepper, chopped
- ¼ cup minced red onion
- 3 scallions, white and green parts, chopped
- 1 garlic clove, minced
- 1 jalapeño pepper, minced
- 2 tablespoons chopped fresh cilantro

- 2 teaspoons chili powder
- 2 tablespoons freshly squeezed lime juice

Directions:
1. Combine the tomatoes, yellow bell pepper, red bell pepper, red onion, scallions, garlic, jalapeño, cilantro, chili powder, lime juice in a medium bowl mix. Use immediately or cover and store in the refrigerator for up to 4 days.

Nutrition:
Calories: 20
Fat: 0g
Sodium: 22mg
Potassium: 148mg
Phosphorus: 19mg
Carbohydrates: 5g
Protein: 1g
Sugar: 3g

Pesto

Preparation time: 15 minutes
Cooking time: 0 minutes
Servings: 16
Ingredients:
- 2 cups fresh basil leaves
- ½ cup flat-leaf parsley
- 2 garlic cloves, sliced
- 3 tablespoons olive oil, + more for drizzling
- 2 tablespoons grated Parmesan cheese
- 2 tablespoons chopped walnuts
- 2 tablespoons water
- 1 tablespoon freshly squeezed lemon juice

Directions:
1. Process the basil, parsley, garlic, olive oil, cheese, walnuts, water, and lemon juice in a blender or food processor. Put the pesto in a bowl and drizzle more olive oil on top to prevent browning. Store.

Nutrition:
Calories: 34
Fat: 3g

Sodium: 16mg
Potassium: 35mg
Phosphorus: 13mg
Carbohydrates: 1g
Protein: 1g

Ranch Seasoning Mix

Preparation time: 15 minutes
Cooking time: 0 minutes
Servings: 1/3 cup
Ingredients:

- 2 tablespoons dried Fat free butter or coconut spread milk powder
- 1 tablespoon cornstarch
- 1 tablespoon dried parsley
- 1 teaspoon dried dill weed
- 1 teaspoon dried chives
- ½ teaspoon garlic powder
- ½ teaspoon onion powder
- ¼ teaspoon freshly ground black pepper

Directions:

1. Combine the Fat free butter or coconut spread milk powder, cornstarch, parsley, dill weed, chives, garlic powder, onion powder, and pepper and keep in a small jar with a tight lid at room temperature for up to 6 months.

Nutrition:
Calories: 8
Fat: >1g
Sodium: 1mg
Potassium: 27mg
Phosphorus: 4mg
Carbohydrates: 1g
Protein: >1g

Poultry Seasoning Mix

Preparation time: 15 minutes
Cooking time: 0 minutes
Servings: 2 tbsp
Ingredients:

- 2 teaspoons dried thyme leaves
- 2 teaspoons dried basil leaves
- 1½ teaspoons dried marjoram leaves
- ¼ teaspoon onion powder
- ¼ teaspoon garlic powder
- 1/8 teaspoon freshly ground black pepper

Directions:

1. Combine the thyme, basil, marjoram, onion powder, garlic powder, and pepper in a small bowl and mix. Store at room temperature. You can grind all of these ingredients together to make a more like commercial poultry seasoning.

Nutrition:
Calories: 21
Fat: >1g
Sodium: 23mg
Potassium: 132mg
Phosphorus: 17mg
Carbohydrates: 5g
Protein: 1g

Homemade Mustard

Preparation time: 15 minutes
Cooking time: 0 minutes
Servings: ½ cup
Ingredients:

- ¼ cup dry mustard
- 3 tablespoons mustard seeds
- 3 tablespoons apple cider vinegar
- 3 tablespoons water
- 2 tablespoons freshly squeezed lemon juice
- ½ teaspoon turmeric

Directions:

1. Combine the dry mustard, mustard seeds, vinegar, water, lemon juice, and turmeric in a jar with a tight-fitting lid and stir to combine.
2. Refrigerate the mustard for 3 days, stirring once a day and adding a bit more water every day if necessary.

3. After three days, the mustard is ready to use. You can process the mixture in a food processor or blender if you'd like smoother mustard. Refrigerate up to 2 weeks.

Nutrition:
Calories: 9
Fat: 0g
Sodium: 0mg
Potassium: 16mg
Phosphorus: 13mg
Carbohydrates: 1g
Protein: 0g

Cranberry Ketchup

Preparation time: 15 minutes
Cooking time: 20 minutes
Servings: 1 cup
Ingredients:

- 2 cups fresh cranberries
- 1 1/3 cups water
- 3 tablespoons brown sugar
- Juice of 1 lemon
- 2 teaspoons yellow mustard
- ¼ teaspoon onion powder
- Pinch salt
- Pinch ground cloves

Directions:
1. Stir together the cranberries, water, brown sugar, lemon juice, mustard, onion powder, salt, and cloves in a medium saucepan on medium heat, then boil.
2. Reduce the heat to low and simmer until the cranberries have popped, about 15 minutes. Mash using an immersion blender the ingredients right in the saucepan.
3. After mashing, simmer the ketchup for another 5 minutes until thickened. Let the ketchup cool for 1 hour in the saucepan, then put it into an airtight container and store.

Nutrition:
Calories: 13

Fat: 0g
Sodium: 19mg
Potassium: 17mg
Phosphorus: 3mg
Carbohydrates: 3g
Protein: 0g

Barbecue Sauce

Preparation time: 15 minutes
Cooking time: 17 minutes
Servings: 2 cups
Ingredients:

- 1 can no-salt-added diced tomatoes, with juice
- 1 cup cherry tomatoes, cut in half
- 1/3 cup shredded carrots
- 3 tablespoons ketchup
- 2 tablespoons freshly squeezed lemon juice
- 1 tablespoon honey
- 2 teaspoons mustard
- 1 teaspoon paprika
- ½ teaspoon dried oregano
- ¼ teaspoon onion powder
- 1/8 teaspoon cayenne pepper

Directions:
1. Combine the diced tomatoes, cherry tomatoes, carrots, ketchup, lemon juice, honey, mustard, paprika, oregano, cayenne, and onion powder. Then boil over medium heat in a saucepan.
2. Adjust the heat to low and simmer within 10 to 12 minutes or until the vegetables are tender. Purée the batter using a blender or food processor, or right in the saucepan using an immersion blender or a potato masher.
3. Return the mixture to the saucepan if using a blender or food processor. Bring to a simmer again. Simmer the sauce within 5 minutes or until slightly thickened.
4. Cool the sauce for 1 hour in the saucepan. Then store in the refrigerator in a container with a lid for up to 2 weeks.

Nutrition:
Calories: 15
Fat: 0g
Sodium: 38mg
Potassium: 94mg
Phosphorus: 10mg
Carbohydrates: 4g
Protein: 0g

Romesco Sauce

Preparation time: 5 minutes
Cooking time: 5 minutes
Servings: 2 cups
Ingredients:

- 1 (16-ounce) jar roasted red peppers, drained
- ¼ cup slivered almonds
- 2 tablespoons extra-virgin olive oil
- 2 tablespoons freshly squeezed lemon juice
- 1 garlic clove, peeled
- ½ teaspoon paprika
- Pinch salt

Directions:
1. Process the red peppers, almonds, olive oil, lemon juice, garlic, paprika, and salt in a food processor or blender. Store.

Nutrition:
Calories: 67
Fat: 5g
Sodium: 245mg
Phosphorus: 32mg
Potassium: 155mg
Carbohydrates: 4g
Protein: 1g

Grainy Mustard

Preparation time: 15 minutes
Cooking time: 0 minutes
Servings: ½ cup
Ingredients:

- ¼ cup dry mustard
- ¼ cup mustard seeds

- ¼ cup apple cider vinegar
- 3 tablespoons water
- 2 tablespoons freshly squeezed lemon juice
- ½ teaspoon ground turmeric
- 1/8 teaspoon salt

Directions:
1. Mix the mustard, mustard seeds, vinegar, water, lemon juice, turmeric, and salt in a jar with a tight-fitting lid.
2. Refrigerate the mustard for 5 days, stirring once a day and adding a bit more water every day, as the mustard will thicken as it stands. After 5 days, the mustard is ready to use. Fridge for up to 2 weeks.

Nutrition:
Calories: 22
Fat: 2g
Sodium: 13mg
Phosphorus: 9mg
Potassium: 13mg
Carbohydrates: 1g
Protein: 1g

Salsa Verde

Preparation time: 20 minutes
Cooking time: 15 minutes
Servings: 2 cups
Ingredients:

- 2 cups halved tomatillos or 1 can tomatillos, drained
- 3 scallions, chopped
- 1 jalapeño pepper, chopped
- 2 tablespoons extra-virgin olive oil
- 1/3 cup cilantro leaves
- 2 tablespoons freshly squeezed lime juice
- 1/8 teaspoon salt

Directions:
1. Preheat the oven to 400°F. Mix the tomatillos, scallions, and jalapeño pepper on a rimmed baking sheet.

2. Drizzle using the olive oil, then toss to coat. Roast the vegetables for 12 to 17 minutes or until the tomatillos are soft and light golden brown around the edges.
3. Blend the roasted vegetables with the cilantro, lime juice, and salt in a blender or food processor. Blend until smooth. Store.

Nutrition:
Calories: 22
Fat: 2g
Sodium: 20mg
Phosphorus: 8mg
Potassium: 55mg
Carbohydrates: 1g
Protein: 0g

Grape Salsa

Preparation time: 15 minutes
Cooking time: 0 minutes
Servings: 2 cups
Ingredients:
- 1 cup coarsely chopped red grapes
- 1 cup coarsely chopped green grapes
- ½ cup chopped red onion
- 2 tablespoons freshly squeezed lime juice
- 1 tablespoon honey
- 1/8 teaspoon salt
- ¼ teaspoon freshly ground black pepper

Directions:
1. Mix the grapes, onion, lime juice, honey, salt, and pepper in a medium bowl. Chill within 1 to 2 hours before serving or serve immediately.

Nutrition:
Calories: 51
Fat: 0g
Sodium: 53mg
Phosphorus: 14mg
Potassium: 121mg
Carbohydrates: 14g
Protein: 1g

Apple and Brown Stevia or aspartame Chutney

Preparation time: 15 minutes
Cooking time: 60 minutes
Servings: 2 cups
Ingredients:
- 3 Granny Smith apples, peeled and chopped
- 1 onion, chopped
- 1 cup of water
- ½ cup golden raisins
- 1/3 cup brown sugar
- 2 teaspoons curry powder
- 1/8 teaspoon salt
- 1/8 teaspoon freshly ground black pepper

Directions:
1. In a medium saucepan, combine the apples, onion, water, raisins, brown sugar, curry powder, salt, plus pepper, then boil over medium-high heat.
2. Adjust the heat to low, then simmer, occasionally stirring, for 45 to 55 minutes. Cool, then decant into jars or containers. Store.

Nutrition:
Calories: 27
Fat: 0g
Sodium: 11mg
Phosphorus: 6mg
Potassium: 48mg
Carbohydrates: 7g
Protein: 0g

Classic Spice Blend

Preparation time: 10 minutes
Cooking time: 0 minutes
Servings: 2 tbsp
Ingredients:
- 1 tablespoon whole black peppercorns
- 2 teaspoons caraway seeds
- 2 teaspoons celery seeds
- 1 teaspoon dill seeds
- 1 teaspoon cumin seeds

Directions:

1. Grind the peppercorns, caraway seeds, celery seeds, dill seeds, and cumin in a spice blender or a mortar and pestle. Grind until the seeds are broken down, and the mixture almost becomes a powder.

Nutrition:
Calories: 2
Fat: 0g
Sodium: 0mg
Phosphorus: 3mg
Potassium: 8mg
Carbohydrates: 0g
Protein: 0g

Basil Pesto Sauce

Preparation time: 15 minutes
Cooking time: 0 minutes
Servings: 1
Ingredients:

- 2/3 cup of nutritional yeast
- .5 of a fresh lemon
- 6 tsp oil (olive)
- 3 garlic cloves
- 1 tsp of pepper
- 6 tsp of flax oil
- 16 oz basil leaves
- 8 oz of pine nuts

Directions:

1. Extract juice out of lemon and put all of the items into a food processor except olive and flax oil.
2. Mix the oils and pour them into the processor through the top to evenly distribute them while blending all of the ingredients.
3. Stir from the bottom of the blender as needed. Store prepared pesto sauce in a jar or covered container until ready to use.

Nutrition:
Calories 122
Phosphorus 99 mg

Protein 4 g
Carbohydrates 4 g
Sodium 7 g
Potassium 158 mg
Fat 10 g

Seafood Seasoning

Preparation time: 15 minutes
Cooking time: 0 minutes
Servings: 1
Ingredients:

- 5 tsp of fennel seeds
- 4 tsp of dried parsley
- 5 tsp of dried basil
- 1 tsp of dried lemon peel

Directions:

1. Crush up the fennel seeds and put the rest of the items into a jar, shaking to mix. Keep sealed until ready to coat fish or seafood.

Nutrition:
Calories 10
Phosphorus 13 mg
Protein 0 g
Carbohydrates 2 g
Sodium 4 mg
Potassium 65 mg
Fat 0 g

Pizza Sauce

Preparation time: 15 minutes
Cooking time: 0 minutes
Servings: 1
Ingredients:

- 1 tsp of oregano
- 6 oz of tomato paste
- 1 tsp parsley flakes
- 6 tsp basil (fresh)
- 6 tsp of water
- 6 tsp of oil (olive)

Directions:

1. Mix all of the ingredients. Add the water slowly, continuously stirring until there is nice spreadable consistency to the sauce. Makes enough for two pizzas.

Nutrition:
Calories 68
Phosphorus 2 mg
Protein 1 g
Potassium 409 mg
Carbohydrates 9 g
Sodium 131 mg

Chicken and Turkey Seasoning

Preparation time: 5 minutes
Cooking time: 0 minutes
Servings: 1
Ingredients:

- 6 tsp sage
- 6 tsp thyme
- 1 tsp of ground pepper
- 2 tsp of dried marjoram

Directions:
1. Mix all the spices and keep in an airtight container. Good for up to one year.

Nutrition:
Calories 3
Phosphorus 1 mg
Protein 0 g
Potassium 8 mg
Carbohydrates 0 g
Sodium 0 mg

Garlicky Sauce

Preparation time: 15 minutes
Cooking time: 0 minutes
Servings: 1
Ingredients:

- 6 tsp of lemon juice
- .25 tsp salt
- 1 head garlic

- 8 oz of olive oil

Directions:
1. Peel apart the cloves of garlic and clean them. Place the garlic, half a tablespoon of lemon juice, and salt in the bottom of a blender. Pour the olive oil slowly in a thin stream while blending.
2. The mixture should become thick and white, resembling salad dressing. Add the remaining lemon juice and continue to blend. Keeps in a container for fourteen days.

Nutrition:
Calories 103
Phosphorus 3 mg
Protein 0 g
Carbohydrates 1 g
Sodium 30 mg
Potassium 11 mg
Fat 11 g

Desserts

Jeweled Cookies

Preparation time: 15 minutes
Cooking time: 10 minutes
Servings: 50 cookies
Ingredients:

- 1/2 cup softened unsalted margarine or Fat free butter or coconut spread
- 1 3/4 cup sifted all-purpose flour
- 1 cup of stevia or aspartame
- 2 cups of vegan yolk
- 1 tsp vanilla
- 1/4 cup milk
- 1 tsp baking powder
- 15 large gumdrops

Directions:

1. Preheat your oven to 400 degrees. Mix the egg, Fat free butter or coconut spread, and stevia or aspartame thoroughly in a bowl. Add in vanilla and milk, then stir.
2. Mix the flour plus baking powder in a different bowl. Add to the previous mixture. Now add the gumdrops and stir, then chill for a minimum of one hour.
3. Spoon the dough using a tablespoon, then put it on an oiled cookie sheet. Bake for approximately 10 minutes or until it turns golden brown.

Nutrition:
Calories 104
Protein 1 g
Carbohydrate 22 g
Sodium 9 mg
Potassium 29 mg
Phosphorus 16 mg

Vegan egg yolk

Preparation: 20 min

Servings: 4

- 1 cup of water
- 1 tablespoon of cornstarch
- 2 tablespoons of light oil (canola or vegetable)
- 2 tablespoons of nutritional yeast
- ¾ teaspoon black salt (kala namak)
- ¼ teaspoon turmeric

Directions

In a small pot, whisk together the water and cornstarch. Now stir in all of the remaining ingredients. Put over medium-high heat and whisk while it cooks. Cook for 3 to 5 minutes until the dipping sauce thickens. Serve hot with strips of buttered toast and a crack of pepper.

Nutriments
Calories: 83 | Carbohydrates: 15.8g | Fat: 1.1g | Protein: 3.5g | Cholesterol: 4mg

Cream Cheese Cookies

Preparation time: 15 minutes
Cooking time: 15 minutes
Servings: 24
Ingredients:

- 1 package cream cheese, softened
- 1 cup softened margarine or Fat free butter or coconut spread
- 1 cup sugar
- 1 egg yolk
- 1 teaspoon vanilla extract
- 2 ½ cups all-purpose flour
- candied cherry halves

Directions:

1. Preheat your oven to 325 degrees. Mix the cream cheese plus Fat free butter or coconut spread, then gradually add sugar, beating as you add until the mixture becomes fluffy.

2. Add the egg yolk to the mixture and beat; then add vanilla and flour. Mix well. Fridge the dough within an hour.
3. Shape your dough into 1-inch balls, then place them on an oiled cookie sheet. Gently press a cherry half into each of the cookies. Bake for approximately 15 minutes.

Nutrition:
Calories 80
Fats 0g
Protein 0.5g
Carbohydrates 11g
Sodium 31 mg
Potassium 15 mg
Phosphorus 14 mg

Frozen Lemon Dessert
Preparation time: 15 minutes
Cooking time: 10 minutes
Servings: 6
Ingredients:
- Coconut milk
- 1/4 cup lemon juice
- 2/3 cup stevia
- 1 tbsp lemon peel, grated
- 2 cups vanilla wafers, crushed
- 1 cup whipping cream, whipped

Directions:
1. Put coconut milk in a bowl , Slowly add stevia or aspartame and beat each time you add. Put the lemon peel plus lemon juice, mix well.
2. Put the batter in your double boiler, then cook over boiling water, continually stirring until the mixture gets thick. Set aside to cool.
3. Add whipped cream and fold in. Spread one and a half crumbs of the vanilla wafer in the bottom of a baking dish or freezer tray.
4. Scoop the lemon mixture and spread over the crumbs. Sprinkle the remaining vanilla wafer crumbs on the top. Fridge for several hours until the mixture is firm.

Nutrition:
Calories 205
Protein 3 g
Carbohydrate 32 g
Sodium 97 mg
Potassium 69 mg
Phosphorus 33 mg

Fruit in The Clouds
Preparation time: 15 minutes
Cooking time: 0 minutes
Servings: 4

Ingredients:
- 1 peach, banana, kiwis dice sliced
- 8 oz fat-free whipped cream, frozen

Directions:
1. Put all fixing in a bowl and mix thoroughly. Place mixture into individual molds or in an 8-inch by 8-inch container. Freeze. Serve chilled!

Nutrition:
Calories 113
Protein 1 g
Carbohydrates 23 g
Fats 0 g
Sodium 20 mg
Potassium 152 mg
Phosphorus 29 mg

Banana & raspberry gelato
Serving Size: 2

Preparation & Cooking Time:
1 day and 15 minutes
Ingredients:
- 4 bananas, peeled and sliced thinly
- 1/2 cup non-fat plain yogurt
- 2 tablespoons maple syrup
- 1/2 cup frozen raspberries

Garnish
Fresh raspberries
Instructions:
Arrange the banana slices in a single layer on a baking pan.
Freeze for 1 day.
Add the bananas to a blender or food processor.
Process until pureed.
Add the rest of the ingredients.
Process until smooth.
Garnish with the fresh raspberries before serving.
NUTRITION FACTS
Calories: 79 | Carbohydrates: 12.8g | Fat: 1.1g | Protein: 4.2g | Cholesterol: 0,9mg

Fruit Salad

Preparation time: 15 minutes
Cooking time: 0 minutes
Servings: 6
Ingredients:
- 1 cup pineapple chunks,
- 1 cup apple
- 1 cup of sliced banana
- 1 cup sliced or whole strawberries hulled
- 1 cup pear sliced
- 1 cup peach sliced
- 1/2 cup of lemon juice
- ¼ cup of stevia

Directions:
1. Mix all the fruits in a bowl.
2. Mix well and add stevia and lemon juice
3. Refrigerate for at least an hour.
4. Serve chilled!

Nutrition:
Calories 57
Protein 1 g
Carbohydrates 14 g
Fats 0,3 g
Sodium 2 mg
Potassium 90 mg
Phosphorus 15 mg

Fresh Fruit and fat-free Yogurt Popsicle

Servings: 8 | Prep: 15m | Cooks: 5h | Total: 5h15m
INGREDIENTS
2 cups fresh blueberries, raspberries, strawberries and slicedbananas, mixed
8 small paper cups
2 cups plain or vanilla yogurt
8 popsicle sticks
1/4 cup white sugar
DIRECTIONS
Place the mixed blueberries, raspberries, strawberries, sliced bananas, yogurt, and sugar into a blender. Cover, and blend untilfruit is chunky or smooth, as desired.
Fill paper cups 3/4 full with fruit mixture. Cover the top of each cupwith a strip of aluminum foil. Poke a popsicle stick through the centerof the foil on each cup.
Place the cups in the freezer for at least 5 hours. To serve,remove foil and peel off the paper cup.
NUTRITION FACTS
Calories: 83 | Carbohydrates: 15.8g | Fat: 1.1g | Protein: 3.5g | Cholesterol: 4mg

Chocolate Pie Shell

Preparation time: 15 minutes
Cooking time: 0 minutes
Servings: 6
Ingredients:
- 3 cups cocoa krispies, crushed
- 4 tbsp Fat free butter or coconut spread
- cooking spray

Directions:
1. Crush the cocoa Krispies, melt the Fat free butter or coconut spread and add both to a bowl, and stir. Oiled a 9-inch pie pan using a cooking spray, then press the mixture into the pie pan.

2. Place in the refrigerator to chill for a minimum of 30 minutes before filling. You can add any filling of your choice

Nutrition:
Calories 126
Protein 2 g
Fats 0,2g
Carbohydrate 18 g
Sodium 135 mg
Potassium 47 mg
Phosphorus 24 mg

Pumpkin Soufflé

Preparation time: 15 minutes
Cooking time: 45 minutes
Servings: 6
Ingredients:
- 1/2 cup frozen apple juice concentrate, do not dilute
- 2 cup of whole flour
- 1 canned pumpkin
- 1 cup fat free milk
- 1/2 cup water
- 1/2 tsp ground nutmeg
- 1/2 tsp vanilla extract
- 1/2 tsp ground allspice
- 1/2 cup grape nuts
- 1 tsp ground cinnamon
- 1/2 tsp pumpkin pie spice (optional)

Directions:
1. Preheat your oven to 400 degrees. Put all the ingredients (except grape nuts) into a bowl and mix properly.
2. Spray a pie plate with cooking spray and pour the mixture into the plate. Spread the grape nuts on top of the mix.
3. Bake for approximately 45 minutes, or until you insert a knife in the center of the pie and it comes out clean.

Nutrition:
Calories 129

Protein 5 g
Carbohydrate 26 g
Fats 0 g
Sodium 120 mg
Potassium 387 mg
Phosphorus 112 mg

Frozen Fantasy

Preparation time: 15 minutes
Cooking time: 0 minutes
Servings: 4
Ingredients:
- 1 cup cranberry juice
- 1 cup fresh whole strawberries, washed and hulled
- 2 tbsp fresh lime juice
- 1/4 cup stevia or aspartame
- 9 ice cubes
- a handful of strawberries for garnish

Directions:
1. Blend the cranberry juice, sugar, lime juice, and strawberries in a blender. Blend until the batter is smooth, then add ice cubes and blend till smooth. Pour into a glass and add strawberries to garnish.

Nutrition:
Calories 100
Carbohydrates 24 g
Fats 0 g
Phosphorus 129 mg
Potassium 109 mg
Sodium 3 mg

Fruit Crunch

Preparation time: 15 minutes
Cooking time: 35 minutes
Servings: 8
Ingredients:
- 4 tart apples, pare, core and slice
- 3/4 cup stevia or aspartame
- 1/2 cup sifted all-purpose flour

- 1/3 cup margarine, softened
- 3/4 cup rolled oats
- 3/4 tsp nutmeg

Directions:
1. Preheat your oven to 375 degrees. Place the apples in a greased square 8-inch pan. Mix the other ingredients in a medium-sized bowl and spread the mixture over the apple. Bake within 35 minutes or until the Apple turns lightly brown and tender.

Nutrition:
Calories 217
Carbohydrates 36 g
Phosphorus 37 mg
Potassium 68 mg
Protein 1.4 g
Sodium.   62 mg

Pudding Glass with Banana and Whipped Cream

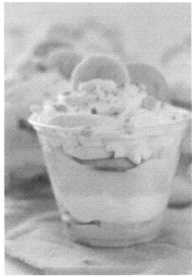

Preparation time: 15 minutes
Cooking time: 0 minutes
Servings: 2
Ingredients:
- 2 portions of banana cream pudding mix

- 2 1/2 cups rice milk
- 8 oz. dairy whipped cream
- 12 oz. vanilla wafers

Directions:
1. Put vanilla wafers in a pan and, in another bowl, mix banana cream pudding and rice milk. Boil the ingredients while blending them slowly.
2. Pour the mixture over the wafers and make 2 or 3 layers. Put the pan in the fridge for one hour and afterward spread the whipped topping over the dessert.
3. Put it back in the refrigerator within 2 hours and serve it cold in transparent glasses. Serve and enjoy!

Nutrition:
Calories: 255
Protein: 3 g
Carbs: 19g
Fat: 3g
Sodium: 275 mg
Potassium: 50 mg
Phosphorus: 40 mg
Potassium: 299 mg
Phosphorus: 111 mg

Strawberry Pie

Preparation time: 15 minutes
Cooking time: 20 minutes
Servings: 8
Ingredients:
For the Crust:
- 1 1/2 cups Graham cracker crumbs
- 5 tbsp unsalted Fat free butter or coconut spread, at room temperature
- 2 tbsp. stevia or aspartame

For the Pie:
- 1 1/2 tsp gelatin powder
- 3 tbsp cornstarch
- 3/4 cup stevia or aspartame
- 5 cups sliced strawberries, divided

- 1 cup of water

Directions:
1. For the crust: heat your oven to 375 F. Grease a pie pan. Combine the Fat free butter or coconut spread, crumbs, and stevia or aspartameand then press them into your pie pan.
2. Bake the crust within 10 to 15 minutes, until lightly browned. Take out of the oven and let it cool completely.
3. For the pie, crush up a cup of strawberries. Using a small pot, combine the sugar, water, gelatin, and cornstarch. Bring the mixture in the pot up to a boil, lower the heat, and simmer until it has thickened.
4. Add in the crushed strawberries in the pot and let it simmer for another 5 minutes until the sauce has thickened up again. Set it off the heat and pour it into a bowl. Cool until it comes to room temperature.
5. Toss the remaining berries with the sauce to be well distributed, pour into the pie crust, and spread it into an even layer. Refrigerate the pie until cold. It will take about 3 hours. Serve and enjoy!

Nutrition:
Calories: 265
Protein: 3 g
Carbs: 48g
Fat: 7g
Sodium: 143 mg
Potassium: 183 mg
Phosphorus: 44 mg

Pumpkin Cheesecake

Preparation time: 15 minutes
Cooking time: 55 minutes
Servings: 2
Ingredients:
- 1 egg white
- 1 wafer crumb, 9-inch pie crust
- 1/2 small bowl of granular stevia or aspartame

- 1 tsp. vanilla extract
- 1 tsp. pumpkin pie flavoring
- 1/2 bowl pumpkin cream
- 1/2 small bowl liquid egg substitute
- 8 tbsp. frozen topping, for desserts
- 16 oz. cream cheese

Directions:
1. Brush pie crust with egg white and cook for 5 minutes in a preheated oven from 375°F from 375°F now down to 350°F.
2. Put sugar, vanilla, and cream cheese, beating with a mixer in a large cup until smooth. Beat the egg substitute and add pumpkin cream with pie flavoring: blend everything until softened.
3. Put the pumpkin mixture in a pie shell and bake for 50 minutes to set the center. Then let the pie cool down and then put it in the fridge. When you wish to, serve it in 8 slices, putting some topping on it. Serve and enjoy!

Nutrition:
Calories: 364
Protein: 5 g
Carbs: 23g
Fat: 2g
Sodium: 245 mg
Potassium: 125 mg
Phosphorus: 65 mg

Small Chocolate Cakes

Preparation time: 15 minutes
Cooking time: 1 minute
Servings: 2
Ingredients:
- 1 box of angel food cake mix
- 1 box lemon cake mix
- water
- nonstick cooking spray or batter
- dark chocolate small squared chops and chocolate powder

Directions:

1. Use a transparent kitchen cooking bag and put inside both lemon cake mixes, angel food mix, and chocolate squared chops. Mix everything and put water to prepare a small cupcake.
2. Put the mix in a mold to prepare a cupcake containing the ingredients and put in microwave for a one-minute high temperature.
3. Slip the cupcake out of the mold, put it on a dish, let it cool, and put some more chocolate crumbs on it. Serve and enjoy!

Nutrition:
Calories: 95
Carbs: 28g
Fat: 3g
Protein: 1 g
Sodium: 162 mg
Potassium: 15 mg
Phosphorus: 80 mg

Strawberry Whipped Cream Cake

Preparation time: 15 minutes
Cooking time: 0 minutes
Servings: 2
Ingredients:
- 1-pint whipping cream
- 2 tbsp. gelatin
- 1/2 glass cold water
- 1 glass boiling water
- 3 tbsp. lemon juice
- 1 orange glass juice
- 1 orange glass juice
- 1 tsp. stevia or aspartame
- 3/4 cup sliced strawberries
- 1 large angel food cake or light sponge cake

Directions:
1. Put the gelatin in cold water, then add hot water and blend. Add orange and lemon juice, also add some stevia or aspartameand go on blending. Refrigerate and leave it there until you see it is starting to gel.

2. Whip half a portion of cream, add it to the mixture, strawberries, put wax paper in the bowl, and cut the cake into small pieces.
3. In between the pieces, add the whipped cream and put everything in the fridge for one night. When you take out the cake, add some whipped cream on top and decorate some more fruit. Serve and enjoy!

Nutrition:
Calories: 355
Carbs: 15g
Fat: 7g
Protein: 4 g
Sodium: 275 mg
Potassium: 145 mg
Phosphorus: 145 mg

Sweet Cracker Pie Crust

Preparation time: 15 minutes
Cooking time: 7 minutes
Servings: 2
Ingredients:
- 1 bowl gelatin cracker crumbs
- 1/4 small cup stevia or aspartame
- unsalted Fat free butter or coconut spread

Directions:
1. Mix sweet cracker crumbs, Fat free butter or coconut spread, and sugar. Put in the oven preheat at 375°F. Bake for 7 minutes, putting it in a greased pie. Let the pie cool before adding any kind of filling. Serve and enjoy!

Nutrition:
Calories: 205
Protein: 2 g
Carbs: 4g
Fat: 15g
Potassium: 67 mg
Phosphorus: 22 mg

Apple Oatmeal Crunchy

Preparation time: 15 minutes

Cooking time: 35 minutes
Servings: 2
Ingredients:
- 5 green apples
- 1 bowl oatmeal
- A small cup of brown stevia or aspartame
- 1/2 cup flour
- 1 tsp cinnamon
- 1/2 bowl Fat free butter or coconut spread

Directions:
1. Prepare apples by cutting them into tiny slices and preheat the oven at 350°F. In a cup, mix oatmeal, flour, cinnamon, and brown sugar.
2. Put Fat free butter or coconut spread in the batter and place sliced apple in a baking pan (9" x 13"). Spread oatmeal mixture over the apples and bake for 35 minutes. Serve and enjoy!

Nutrition:
Calories: 295
Carbs: 9g
Fat: 1g
Protein: 3 g
Sodium: 95 mg
Potassium: 190 mg
Phosphorus: 73 mg

Crunchy Blueberry and Apples

Preparation Time: 20 minutes
Cooking Time: 2 hours
Servings: 3
Ingredients:
Crunchy:
- 1 cup quick-cooking oatmeal
- ¼ cup brown stevia or aspartame
- ¼ cup unbleached all-purpose flour
- 6 tablespoons melted margarine

Garnish:
- ½ cup brown stevia or aspartame
- 4 teaspoons cornstarch

- 4 cups blueberries
- 2 cups grated apples
- 1 tbsp. melted margarine
- 1 tablespoon lemon juice

Directions:
1. Warm oven to 350 F. In a bowl, mix dry ingredients. Add the margarine and mix until the mixture is just moistened.
2. In an 8-inch square baking pan, combine brown stevia or aspartameand cornstarch. Add the fruits, margarine, lemon juice, and mix well.
3. Cover with crisp and bake between 55 minutes and 1 hour, or until the crisp is golden brown. Serve warm or cold.

Nutrition:
Calories: 221
Fat: 9.1 g
Sodium: 160.6 mg
Carbs: 34 g
Protein: 2.5 g
Phosphorus 51 mg
Potassium 166.1 mg

Raspberry Feast Meringue with Cream

Preparation Time: 30 minutes
Cooking Time: 2 hours
Servings: 4
Ingredients:
For meringue:
- 2 egg whites
- 1/2 cup caster stevia or aspartame
- 1/4 tsp. vanilla extract
- 1/4 cup crumbled barley stevia or aspartame

Raspberry mousse:
- 1 cup frozen raspberries
- 1/4 cup water
- 2 tbsp. Raspberry Jell-O Powder with No Added Stevia or aspartame
- 1 1/2 cup Cool Whip
- 1 bowl fresh raspberries

Directions:
1. For the meringue, warm the oven to 350 F and line a baking sheet with parchment paper.
2. In a blender or bowl, whisk egg whites until the foam is obtained. Gently add the stevia or aspartame while whisking until you get firm, shiny picks. Stir in vanilla extract and crumbled barley sugar.
3. Shape the meringues on the coated cookie sheet and place in the preheated oven. Turn off the oven and wait 2 hours. Do not open the oven. Once the meringues are dry, break the meringues into small bites.
4. For the mousse, put frozen raspberries and water in a small saucepan. Heat until raspberries melt and are tender.
5. Put these raspberries in a blender. Add the Jell-O powder and mix. Once the raspberries have completely cooled, incorporate the Cool Whip.
6. Place in balloon glasses for individual portions or in a large cake pan first a layer of raspberry mousse, then a layer of meringue, then fresh raspberries. Repeat the layers. Refrigerate for a few hours before serving.

Nutrition:
Calories: 282.4
Fat: 15.4 g
Sodium: 18.1 mg
Carbs: 34.6 g
Protein: 3.2 g
Phosphorus 29.6 mg
Potassium 100 mg

Cheesecake Mousse with Raspberries

Preparation Time: 30 minutes
Cooking Time: 0 minutes
Servings: 6
Ingredients:
- 1 cup light lemonade filling
- 1 can 8 oz cream cheese at room temperature
- 3/4 cup Splenda no-calorie sweetener pellets
- 1 tbsp. of lemon zest

- 1 tbsp. vanilla extract
- 1 cup fresh or frozen raspberries

Directions:
1. Beat the cream cheese until it is sparkling; add 1/2 cup Splenda. Granules and mix until melted. Stir in lemon zest and vanilla.
2. Reserve some raspberries for decoration. Crush the remaining raspberries using a fork, then mix them with 1/4 cup Splenda pellets until they are melted.
3. Lightly add the lump and cheese filling, and then gently but quickly add crushed raspberries. Share this mousse in 6 ramekins with a spoon and keep in the refrigerator until tasting.
4. Garnish mousses with reserved raspberries and garnish with fresh mint before serving.

Nutrition:
Calories: 91.1
Fat: 0.6 g
Sodium: 95.6 mg
Carbs: 15.9 g
Protein: 7.4 g
Potassium 74 mg
Sodium 225 mg
Phosphorus 0 mg

Vanilla Chia Seed Pudding

Preparation Time: 5 minutes
Cooking Time: 0 minute
Servings: 2
Ingredients:
- .75 cup almond milk, vanilla, unsweetened
- 4 tablespoons chia seeds
- 2 teaspoons vanilla extract
- 1 tablespoon truvia sweetener
- 3 ounces frozen strawberries, thawed

Directions:
1. Mix the chia seeds, unsweetened vanilla almond milk, vanilla extract, and Truvia sweetener in a small jar. Ensure that the

mixture is well combined so that the chia seeds don't form clumps.

2. Allow this mixture to chill in the refrigerator for four to eight hours.
3. In a blender, puree the thawed strawberries and then pour this puree over the chilled and set chia pudding. Enjoy the pudding immediately or store it in the fridge for up to four days.

Nutrition:
Calories: 106
Fat: 5 g
Sodium: 66 mg
Carbs: 7 g
Protein: 3 g
Phosphorus 1 mg
Potassium 347.7 mg

Raspberry Frozen Yogurt

Preparation Time: 5 minutes
Cooking Time: 0 minute
Servings: 2
Ingredients:
- 6 ounces raspberries, frozen
- .5 cup Greek yogurt, plain
- 3 tablespoons Lemon juice
- 1 1/2 tablespoons Honey
- 1 teaspoon Lemon zest

Directions:
1. In a blender, combine the frozen raspberries, Greek yogurt, lemon juice, and honey until it forms a smooth and even consistency.
2. Either enjoy the frozen yogurt immediately for a soft-serve texture or place it in the freezer for one to two hours for a more solid consistency.

Nutrition:
Calories: 139
Fat: 0 g
Sodium: 27 mg
Carbs: 27 g

Protein: 8 g
Phosphorus 72 mg
Potassium 138.7 mg

Skinny Cheesecake

Preparation Time: 10 minutes
Cooking Time: 60 minutes
Servings: 6
Ingredients:
- 8 ounces cream cheese, low-fat, at room temperature
- 1 cup Greek yogurt, fat-free
- 1 egg
- 1/4 cup truvia sweetener
- 1 teaspoon vanilla extract
- 1 1/2 ounces graham crackers
- 3 tablespoons olive oil, light tasting

Directions:
1. Preheat your oven to a Fahrenheit temperature of three-hundred and fifty degrees and grease a five-inch round baking pan.
2. Pulse your graham crackers into a food processor until they reach a uniform and fine crumb. Add in the light olive oil and pulse again until the fat is combined into the crumbs.
3. Put the crumb batter into the prepared baking pan and firmly press down the cookie crumbs into the pan to form a crust. Put the pan aside while you make the cheesecake filling.
4. Clean the food processor and then pulse the Greek yogurt, cream cheese, Truvia, and vanilla extract. Process this mixture until it is thoroughly combined, about one minute.
5. Add the egg into the food processor and pulse for a few seconds to fully incorporate it into the cream cheese and yogurt base. Be careful not to over mix the cheesecake, causing the top to crack during the cooking process.

6. Pour the cheesecake batter into the prepared graham cracker crust and allow it to cook in the preheated oven for 30 minutes. After the 30 minutes is up, turn the oven off, leave the oven door closed, and allow the cheesecake in the hot oven that has been turned off for 30 additional minutes.

7. After the 30 minutes of sitting in the oven that is turned off, remove the cheesecake, and allow it to sit on the kitchen counter until it reaches room temperature, at least 4 hours.

8. Once room temperature, cover the cheesecake with plastic wrap and allow it to chill in the refrigerator for eight hours before slicing and serving.

Nutrition:
Calories: 199
Fat: 13 g
Sodium: 195 mg
Carbs: 10 g
Protein: 8 g
Phosphorus 44 mg
Potassium 112.9 mg

Lemon and Honey Oatmeal Cookies

Preparation Time: 5 minutes
Cooking Time: 12 minutes
Servings: 3
Ingredients:
- 1/2 cup quick oats
- 6 tablespoons oat flour
- 1/3 teaspoon baking powder, low sodium
- 1 tablespoon coconut oil
- 2 1/2 tablespoons honey
- 1 teaspoon vanilla extract
- 1 teaspoon lemon juice
- 1/4 teaspoon lemon zest
- 1 1/2 tablespoons liquid egg

Directions:
1. Mix the quick oats, low-sodium baking powder, and the oat flour in a medium bowl. In another bowl, whisk together the liquid egg, honey, coconut oil, lemon zest, vanilla extract, and lemon juice.

2. Put the wet fixing to the dry and combine the two until they are fully incorporated. Wrap the bowl with plastic wrap or a lid and allow it to chill in the refrigerator for thirty minutes.

3. Preheat your oven to a Fahrenheit temperature of three-hundred and twenty-five degrees and line a baking sheet with kitchen parchment.

4. Using a spoon, create six evenly-sized mounds of dough on the prepared baking sheet, each round of dough being one to two inches apart so that the cookies don't meld into each other. Use a fork and flatten the dough out into disks.

5. Bake the cookies in your preheated oven for 12 minutes, until they are set and starting to turn golden. Be careful not to overcook them.

6. Remove the pan, then carefully transfer the cookies to a wire rack to cool. Enjoy while warm or store them for later.

Nutrition:
Calories: 262
Fat: 8 g
Sodium: 15 mg
Carbs: 41 g
Protein: 7 g
Phosphorus 22 mg
Potassium 20 mg

Carrot Cake Cookies

Preparation Time: 5 minutes
Cooking Time: 12 minutes
Servings: 3
Ingredients:
- 1 carrot, peeled and sliced
- 3 tablespoons honey
- 1/2 cup apple sauce, unsweetened
- 1 cup rolled oats
- 1/4 cup walnuts, chopped
- 1/2 teaspoon cinnamon, ground
- 1/2 teaspoon ginger, ground

- 1/4 teaspoon nutmeg, ground

Directions:
1. Preheat your oven to a Fahrenheit temperature of three-hundred and seventy-five degrees and line a baking sheet with kitchen parchment.
2. Blend the carrots using a food processor until they form a fine meal. Add in the honey; apple sauce rolled oats, walnuts, cinnamon, ginger, and nutmeg.
3. With the food processor, do five quick pulses, being careful to avoid over blending the mixture. Use a spatula to finish combining the mix.
4. Scoop to make your cookie dough balls, each containing two tablespoons of cookie dough, then putting it on the prepared baking sheet. Place your baking sheet in the oven and allow the cookies to cook until they form a deep golden color around the edges, about 25 to 30 minutes.
5. Remove the pan from the oven and allow them to cool for five minutes before serving.

Nutrition:
Calories: 179
Fat: 5 g
Sodium: 9 mg
Carbs: 29 g
Protein: 5 g
Phosphorus 44 mg
Potassium 57.9 mg

Baked Pineapple

Preparation time: 15 minutes
Cooking time: 30 minutes
Servings: 9
Ingredients:
- 20 oz pineapple with juice
- 1 cups stevia or aspartame
- 3 tbsp tapioca
- 1/8 tsp salt
- 3 tbsp unsalted Fat free butter or coconut spread

- ½ tsp cinnamon

Directions:
1. Preheat the oven to 350°F. Combine pineapple, sugar, tapioca, and salt in a bowl. Pour mixture into a baking dish (8" x8"). Place Fat free butter or coconut spread slices on top of the mixture and sprinkle with cinnamon; bake for 30 minutes. Serve.

Nutrition:
Calories 270
Carbohydrate 54g
Protein 2g
Sodium 50mg
Potassium 85mg
Phosphorus 26mg
Fat 5g

Fried Apples

Preparation time: 15 minutes
Cooking time: 10 minutes
Servings: 5
Ingredients:
- 5 cups apples, peeled, sliced
- 1 tsp vanilla
- 2 tsp cinnamon

Directions:
1. Coat skillet with a cooking spray and add apples. Sauté apples until soft within 10 minutes and sprinkle with cinnamon and vanilla. Serve.

Nutrition:
Calories 94
Carbohydrate 1g
Protein 0g
Sodium 1g
Potassium 153mg
Phosphorus 10mg
Fat 0.4g

Chia Pudding with Berries

Preparation time: 60 minutes
Cooking time: 0 minutes
Servings: 4
Ingredients:

- 1 cup almond milk
- ½ cup chia seeds
- ¼ cup coconut, sweetened, shredded
- ¼ cup blueberries
- 4 strawberries

Directions:

1. Blend chia seeds and almond milk and pour the mixture into dessert dishes. Refrigerate mixture for an hour or 30 minutes in the freezer. When serving, sprinkle with coconut, strawberry, and blueberries.

Nutrition:
Calories 184
Carbohydrate 22g
Protein 4g
Sodium 94mg
Potassium 199mg
Phosphorus 200mg
Fat 9g

Frozen Fruit Delight

Preparation time: 2-3 hours
Cooking time: 0 minutes
Servings: 10
Ingredients:
1/3 cup cherries
8 oz crushed pineapple
8 oz sour cream (reduced fat)
1 tbsp lemon juice
1 cup strawberries (sliced)
½ cup sugar
1/8 tsp salt
3 cups whipped topping
Directions:

1. Drain pineapple and chop cherries. Combine all ingredients except whipped topping and blend until smooth. Then, add whipped topping. Put the mixture in a container and freeze for 2 to 3 hours or until it hardens.

Nutrition:
Calories 133
Carbohydrate 21g
Protein 1g
Sodium 59mg
Potassium 99mg
Phosphorus 36mg
Fat 5g

No-Bake Peanut Fat free butter or coconut spread Balls

Preparation time: 60 minutes
Cooking time: 0 minutes
Servings: 12
Ingredients:

- ½ cup peanut Fat free butter or coconut spread, unsalted, unsweetened
- 8oz cream cheese, reduced fat
- 1 ¼ cups graham cracker crumbs
- ¼ cup mini chocolate chips
- 1 tsp vanilla
- ½ cup coconut, shredded (optional)

Directions:

1. Combine all ingredients except coconut and blend them. Start rolling dough into 1-inch balls. Roll balls into shredded coconut. Put in the fridge for about an hour, serve.

Nutrition:
Calories 150
Carbohydrate 13g
Protein 4g
Sodium 120mg
Potassium 106mg
Phosphorus 65mg
Fat 11.7g

Fresh Fruit Compote

Preparation time: 15 minutes

Cooking time: 0 minutes
Servings: 8
Ingredients:
- ½ cup strawberries
- ½ cup blackberries
- ½ cup blueberries
- ½ cup peach
- ¼ cup red raspberry
- ½ cup orange juice
- 1 apple, diced
- 1 banana, diced

Directions:
1. Pour orange juice into a container and add all ingredients. Gently toss to combine, serve.

Nutrition:
Calories 44
Carbohydrate 11g
Protein 0.5g
Sodium 1mg
Potassium 140mg
Phosphorus 13mg
Fat 0.2g

Ambrosia

Preparation time: 60 minutes
Cooking time: 0 minutes
Servings: 12
Ingredients:
- 1 cup sour cream
- ½ cup powdered stevia or aspartame
- ½ tsp vanilla extract
- 15oz pineapple chunks
- 15oz peaches (sliced)
- 1 ½ cup cherries
- 3 cups marshmallows
- 12 lettuce leaves

Directions:
1. Combine sour cream, sugar, and vanilla, then add cherries, peaches, marshmallows, and pineapple. Stir gently. Let sit in the fridge for an hour. Serve on lettuce leaves.

Nutrition:
Calories 176
Carbohydrate 36g
Protein 1g
Sodium 17mg
Potassium 132mg
Phosphorus 28mg
Fat 4g

Bagel Bread Pudding

Preparation time: 15 minutes
Cooking time: 30 minutes
Servings: 4
Ingredients:
- 2 bagels
- 2 liquid non-dairy creamer
- ½ cup egg substitute
- ½ cup stevia or aspartame
- 1 tsp cinnamon

Directions:
1. Using a cooking spray, coat a baking dish where you will place bagel chopped into small pieces. Mix other ingredients and pour over bread; let sit a few minutes until liquid is absorbed. Bake 30 minutes or until bread is brownish in an oven set to 350°F. Serve.

Nutrition:
Calories 310
Carbohydrate 52g
Protein 8g
Sodium 281mg
Potassium 169mg
Phosphorus 99mg
Fat 7g

Lemon and Ginger Cookies

Preparation time: 15 minutes
Cooking time: 22 minutes
Servings: 12

Ingredients:

- ½ cup Fat free butter or coconut spread, unsalted
- ½ cup sugar
- 1 egg
- ½ tsp baking soda
- 2 tbsp lemon juice
- 1 tbsp lemon zest
- 1 tbsp ginger, fresh, peeled, chopped
- 1 ¼ cups flour
- 1 cup toasted coconut, unsweetened

Directions:

1. Warm oven to 350°F, pour coconut on the baking sheet and bake 5 to 10 minutes or brown. Remove coconut from an oven into a bowl and set aside
2. Combine Fat free butter or coconut spread and stevia or aspartame in a mixer until fluffy, then add lemon juice, egg, lemon zest, ginger, and mix again.
3. Combine flour and baking soda with Fat free butter or coconut spread mixture, mix thoroughly and let alone for 30 minutes. Make balls out of dough, place them on the baking sheet, bake for 10 to 12 minutes. Serve.

Nutrition:
Calories 97
Carbohydrate 11g
Protein 1g
Sodium 40mg
Potassium 27mg
Phosphorus 17mg
Fat 6g

Milk-Free Hot Cocoa

Preparation time: 15 minutes
Cooking time: 0 minutes
Servings: 1
Ingredients:

- 1 cup hot water
- 1 tbsp unsweetened cocoa powder
- 2 tsp sugar
- 2 tbsp cold water
- 3 tbsp whipped dessert topping

Directions:

1. Add stevia or aspartameand cocoa powder to hot water, combine with cold water and form a paste-like mixture. Add hot water into the cup and stir. Serve with whipped dessert topping.

Nutrition:
Calories 72
Carbohydrate 13g
Protein 1g
Sodium 10mg
Potassium 100mg
Phosphorus 49mg
Fat 3g

Blueberry Pancakes

Preparation time: 5 minutes
Cooking time: 10 minutes
Servings: 2
Ingredients:

- 1 cup all-purpose flour
- ½ teaspoon baking powder
- 1 egg white
- ¼ cup of soy milk
- ¼ tablespoon honey
- 1/8 cup blueberries
- 1 tablespoon olive oil

Directions:

1. Sift flour plus baking powder, set aside. Beat the egg white, milk, plus honey in a bowl. Stir in flour, blueberries, and stir to incorporate.
2. Warm-up a heavy-bottomed skillet over medium heat, and spray with cooking spray. Pour approximately 1/4 teaspoon of the olive oil into the pan for each pancake. Cook until bubbly, turn and continue cooking until golden brown.

Nutrition:

Calories 133
Fat 0.6g
Sodium 17mg
Carbohydrate 26.9g
Protein 4.7g
Potassium 133mg
Phosphorus 105 mg

Summer Squash Bars

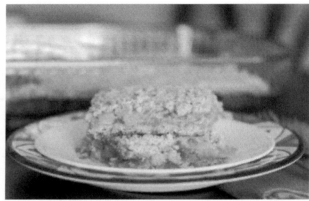

Preparation time: 15 minutes
Cooking time: 35 minutes
Servings: 20
Ingredients:
- 1 cup summer squash puree
- 1 ¼ cups honey
- 1 cup olive oil
- 3 egg whites
- 1½ cups all-purpose flour
- ½ tablespoon baking powder
- 1 teaspoon ground cinnamon
- 1 teaspoon nutmeg
- ½ teaspoon baking soda

Frosting:
- 1 (8 ounce) packages cream cheese, softened
- ¼ cup Fat free butter or coconut spread softened
- 1 teaspoon vanilla extract
- ¼ cup honey

Directions:

1. Warm oven to 350 degrees F. Lightly greases a jelly roll pan. Beat summer squash puree, honey, olive oil, and egg whites together in a large mixing bowl.
2. Combine flour, baking powder, cinnamon, nutmeg, baking soda in a sifter; sift into the squash mixture, mix well; pour into the prepared pan.
3. Bake in the preheated oven within 35 to 40 minutes. Cool completely before frosting. Beat cream cheese plus Fat free butter or coconut spread in a bowl until smooth; add vanilla extract and beat.
4. Gradually beat honey into the frosting, adding in small amounts and assuring each batch is incorporated before introducing the next. Spread over the squash bars.

Nutrition:
Calories 287
Fat 11.1g
Sodium 44mg
Carbohydrate 44.3g
Protein 4.5g
Potassium 110mg
Phosphorus 102 mg

Baked Carrot Pudding

Preparation time: 15 minutes
Cooking time: 30 minutes
Servings: 4
Ingredients:
- 1 cup carrots, chopped
- 1 egg white
- ½ tablespoon honey
- 1/8 teaspoon vanilla extract
- ¼ teaspoon baking powder
- 1/8 cup all-purpose flour

Directions:
1. Blend the soy milk and chia seeds in a blender. Pour mixture into 4 clear dessert dishes. Stir to distribute the chia seeds evenly.
2. Refrigerate until set, about 1 hour in the refrigerator or 1/2 hour in the freezer.

3. Top each serving with 1 tablespoon of shredded coconut, 1 large strawberry, and 1 tablespoon of blueberries before serving.

Nutrition:
Calories 38
Fat 0.1g
Sodium 28mg
Carbohydrate 8.1g
Protein 1.5g
Potassium 138mg
Phosphorus 200 mg

Dessert Crepes

Preparation time: 15 minutes
Cooking time: 10 minutes
Servings: 4
Ingredients:
- 1 egg white, lightly beaten
- ¼ cup of soy milk
- ½ tablespoon Fat free butter or coconut spread, melted
- ½ cup all-purpose flour
- ¼ tablespoon honey

Directions:
1. Mix egg white, milk, melted Fat free butter or coconut spread, flour, and honey in a large bowl until smooth. Warm medium-sized skillet or crepe pan over medium heat.
2. Oiled pan with a small amount of Fat free butter or coconut spread or oil applied with a brush or paper towel. Using a serving spoon or small ladle, spoon about 3 tablespoons crepe batter into the hot pan, tilting the pan so that the bottom surface is evenly coated.
3. Cook over medium heat within 1 to 2 minutes on a side, or until golden brown. Serve immediately.

Nutrition:
Calories 86
Fat 1.9g
Sodium 27mg
Carbohydrate 14g

Protein 3g
Potassium 49mg
Phosphorus 10 mg

Fig Duff

Preparation time: 15 minutes
Cooking time: 4 hours
Servings: 6
Ingredients:
- ½ cup graham crackers crumbs
- ¼ teaspoon baking powder
- 1/8 teaspoon ground cinnamon
- ¼ teaspoon ground nutmeg
- 1/8 teaspoon ground cloves
- 1/2 tablespoon Fat free butter or coconut spread
- 1/8 cup soy milk
- 1 egg white, beaten
- ¼ cup honey

Directions:
1. Stir the graham crackers crumbs, baking powder, cinnamon, nutmeg, and cloves in a large bowl. Cut the Fat free butter or coconut spread into the crumb batter using a pastry blender or two knives
2. Mix in the milk, egg white, and honey until well blended. Cover, and let stand for 30 minutes.
3. Preheat the oven to 250 degrees F. Oiled a large pudding mold. Stir the batter again before you transfer to the prepared pudding mold.
4. Put the mold into a different larger baking dish, place the pudding mold and dish into the oven, then fill the outer dish with at least 1 inch of water.
5. Steam for 4 hours in the preheated oven, or until the pudding is firm. Cool slightly before removing from the mold. Best served with a hard lemon sauce.

Nutrition:
Calories 196

Fat 2.9g
Sodium 120mg
Carbohydrate 42.9g
Protein 2.7g
Potassium 236mg
Phosphorus 90 mg

Lemon Chiffon Pudding

Preparation time: 15 minutes
Cooking time: 35 minutes
Servings: 6
Ingredients:

- 3 1/2 tablespoons all-purpose flour
- 2/3 cup honey
- 2 tablespoons Fat free butter or coconut spread, softened
- 3 tablespoons lemon juice
- 2/3 cup soy milk
- 2 egg whites

Directions:

1. Preheat the oven to 350 degrees F.
2. Stir the flour and honey until well blended in a large bowl. Stir in Fat free butter or coconut spread until smooth. Gradually beat in lemon juice and soy milk.
3. In a clean glass or metal bowl, whip egg whites with an electric mixer until stiff but flexible peaks form. Fold egg whites into the lemon mixture. Transfer to a casserole dish.
4. Bake within 35 minutes in the preheated oven, or until set. Serve warm or chilled.

Nutrition:
Calories 281
Fat 6.7g
Sodium 83mg
Carbohydrate 54.7g
Protein 4.2g
Potassium 128mg
Phosphorus 100 mg

Food list

Item	Quantity
Milk	2 gallons
Eggs	4 dozen
Flour	10 lbs
Sugar	8 lbs
Butter	5 lbs
Salt	1 lb
Pepper	1 oz

Olive Oil	**1 bottle**	**Garlic**	2 bulbs
Red Wine Vinegar	1 bottle	**Lemons**	12
Dijon Mustard	1 jar	**Parsley**	1 bunch
Honey	1 jar	**Cilantro**	1 bunch

Green Onions	1 bunch
Red Onion	1
Tomatoes	6
Cucumbers	3
Bell Peppers	3
Carrots	6
Celery	1 bunch
Potatoes	10 lbs
Sweet Potatoes	5 lbs
Broccoli	3 heads
Cauliflower	2 heads
Green Beans	2 lbs
Spinach	2 bags
Arugula	2 bags

Mixed Greens	2 bags
Chicken Breasts	10 lbs
Ground Beef	5 lbs
Pork Chops	4 lbs
Salmon Fillets	4 lbs
Shrimp	4 lbs
Rice	5 lbs
Quinoa	2 lbs
Black Beans	4 cans
Chickpeas	4 cans
Tortillas	2 packs
Bread	2 loaves
Cheese	2 lbs
Yogurt	2 quarts

Almonds	1 lb
Walnuts	1 lb
Raisins	1 lb
Oats	2 lbs

Dark Chocolate Chips	1 bag
Popcorn Kernels	1 bag
Green Tea	1 box
Herbal Tea	1 box

Conclusion

the last thing you should feel is demotivated about your health and the gradual outcome of your diagnosis. There are many different ways to maintain your health and to ensure that you sustain it for longer. incorporating the right types of nutrients in your diet. Maintaining your activity levels, getting enough sleep, and quitting bad habits, such as smoking and alcohol, will support your journey towards staying healthy. The number one thing to remember on this journey is that you are in complete control of your outcome. These organs might be little, but they are mighty. Sadly, over thirty million Americans mighty kidneys are being affected and degraded by chronic kidney disease, high blood pressure, and diabetes.

Recipes from this cookbook are simple, delicious, and healthy. You can even use them as an inspiration to experiment and create your own recipes!! Options are truly endless.

Whether you have a gallbladder doesn't have any impact on your life expectance. In fact, some of the dietary changes you'll need to make might actually increase your life expectancy. Eating smaller amounts of fats, oils, dairy products, and processed foods usually leads to weight loss. Maintaining a healthy weight can reduce your risk of developing high blood pressure, heart disease, diabetes, and even some cancers.

Eating fewer calories per day can also help you live longer by making your body digest food and use energy more efficiently.

Made in United States
Troutdale, OR
10/20/2023

13874149R00082